Néré St-A

The Politics

of Madness

Translated by Ellen Garmaise and
Robert Chodos

Formac Publishing Company Limited
Halifax, Nova Scotia

PRINTED IN CANADA

Originally published as Folie et oppression
© 1985 Les Editions d'Acadie Ltée, Moncton, New Brunswick

Canadian Cataloguing in Publication Data

St-Amand, Néré,
The Politics of Madness
Translation of: Folie et oppression.
Bibliography: p. 167

ISBN 0-88780-060-2

1. Psychiatric hospitals — New Brunswick —
Sociological aspects. 2. Mentally ill — New
Brunswick. 3. Mental health — New Brunswick.
4. Minorities — Mental health services — New
Brunswick. I. Title.

RC448.N32S7213 1987   362.2'1'09715   C87-094777-X

Formac Publishing
5359 Inglis Street
Halifax, Nova Scotia   B3H 1J4

The Politics
of Madness

To those who see madness in another light

and

*To Lise, Julie and François, for their
patience and understanding*

CONTENTS

LIST OF FIGURES

LIST OF TABLES

Introduction

*If they keep me in a
psychiatric institution
much longer, I'm going to
go crazy!*

— An inmate

The year is 1918. A teenager of Irish origin from the Saint John area, going through a mildly difficult adolescence, is committed to the Provincial Hospital in Saint John, the only psychiatric institution in New Brunswick at that time. In 1982 she is still there. Being a psychiatric patient has virtually become her life's work.

The year is 1981. An Acadian from Kent County is an inmate in the same hospital. When a family member asks that he be released, the hospital director replies that "the treatment program has not been completed yet; when it is, we will certainly let you know." This man has already been there for thirty-seven years; he was admitted in 1944.

These real-life examples immediately raise a series of questions. Why are there psychiatric institutions? Who uses them? What client groups do they serve? Statistics show that the rate of readmission is 65 per cent — doesn't this cast doubt on the kind of treatment used? Moreover, is it acceptable that the goals and structures of psychiatric institutions, indeed their very conception, should have changed so little over the last fifty years?

This study was designed to deal with these concerns and questions about psychiatric institutions. Specifically, it examines the role currently played by these institutions in New Brunswick. The study's working hypotheses involve the relationship between confinement in psychiatric institutions, ethnic origin, and industrialization. Industrial centres were the first places to "organize madness," to use Michel Foucault's expression; with the industrial revolution, laws and institutions for the treatment of the mentally ill developed rapidly in both Europe and America. Hence, as a starting point, this study will examine the relationship between confinement in psychiatric institutions and industrialization. In addition, a number of ethnic groups live in New Brunswick. We will look at how each of these groups sees mental health, and at how the dominated groups — especially the Acadians — react to political-medical oppression as manifested in psychiatric institutions.

A regime has at its disposal a variety of instruments, some more subtle than others, for maintaining order and keeping deviants in their place. The deportation of the Acadians in 1755 was one way of handling the problem. Could psychiatric institutions be a new form of oppression? Are people who refuse to conform to the prevailing social order, and are treated as deviants as a result, subjected to a new kind of "deportation"? In fact, who is psychiatrically normal and who is not? Are there culturally-defined rules governing psychiatric deviance? These questions underlie the study's second working hypothesis, which posits a relationship between ethnicity and mental health. In short, who has power? Who lays down the rules of the game? What about ethnic groups that have no power, and little say in defining laws and policies developed by members of other groups with a different way of thinking — what role do they play?

Medicine, as an organized discipline with the power to diagnose people, decides that a person is mentally ill and puts him or her in the care of an institution created to "cure" the illness. It should be noted that in most cases the individual has not asked to be admitted or treated, and, in New Brunswick today, admission and treatment often take place against the individual's will. In 64 per cent of cases, admission to a psychiatric institution is involuntary; for Acadians, the figure is more than 70 per cent. Individuals do not define their illness: rather, as Roger Bastide has noted, the "norm" decides that they are ill and demands that they be treated.

Once the individual is institutionalized, the psychiatric mechanism takes over from the one that defined the norm. In official documents and speeches, individual and community well-being is said to be the basic goal of these mechanisms. Presenting its official philosophy, the New Brunswick Department of Health* said that "mental health services must be universal and accessible and must meet the needs of the community." In reality, however, is the system in question not a form of oppression imposed by those in power, who use psychiatric institutions and other links in the chain such as doctors and health-care and social-service professionals to maintain their control? All these agents help justify the existence of psychiatric institutions, their practices and their policy of confinement.

Even dominant groups have their outcasts: people they consider ill and outside the norm and therefore want to have treated. But oppressed groups — the Acadians in this study — suffer a double oppression, of which regional disparity, the disadvantages faced by minorities, and the

---

* Now called the Department of Health and Social Services.

form of treatment they are subjected to are all reflections. Through its institutions, the state attempts to make society uniform by homogenizing all groups and individuals. More or less consciously, ethnic groups are manipulated so that they can be dominated and made to submit to the established order and to the system of production on which that order is based. In looking at the history of mental health, will we see this same tendency? This question suggests the possibility of defining mental illness in social rather than psychiatric terms. By introducing cultural specificities as a dimension of our study, we may be able to glimpse the historical and cultural dimensions of mental illness. In short, this study will attempt to assess psychiatric practices in terms of their results, and not in terms of the views of experts.

In order to test these working hypotheses, three approaches have been used. These approaches are sketched briefly here and are explained more fully further on. Throughout the study, reference is made to individual histories. These histories are drawn from the files of 585 individuals admitted to psychiatric institutions between 1956 and 1981, which constitute the sample used for this part of the research. These first-hand accounts are useful in assessing the effects of psychiatric practices on the lives of the individuals concerned. In addition to this anecdotal approach, a statistical analysis of the data contained in the files of the 585 individuals was carried out. Finally, in an attempt to elicit public opinion on the subject of mental health, I conducted a series of interviews. These three approaches complement one another and help provide a way of looking at madness, a portrait of the psychiatric "patient," and a picture of the kinds of treatment used in the mental health system. The stories of particular individuals or groups are not presented as isolated situations, removed from history, social dynamics and the overall contradictions of society. Illness is a message that can be decoded only in the context of the institutions that produce it. We are thus engaged in an inductive process, inseparable from an awareness of the social context that is essential in fleshing out the study of any structure.

The key element in this methodology is its concentration on oppression as the source of the production and reproduction of illness. If this element is ignored, researchers can be come obsessed with symptoms and see themselves as missionaries trying to solve individual problems in isolation from the social issues involved.

1

A History of Inequality: Some Highlights

We Loyalists were an educated group of people. When we came to Canada, we brought our culture with us; the Acadians were more backward.

— An interviewee

If we were right in saying that gods have no use for falsehood and it is useful to mankind only in the way of a medicine, obviously a medicine should be handled by no one but a physician. ... If anyone, then, is to practice deception, either on the country's enemies or on its citizens, it must be the Rulers of the commonwealth, acting for its benefit; no one else may meddle with this privilege. For a private person to mislead such Rulers we shall declare to be a worse offence than for a patient to mislead his doctor.

— Plato[1]

The coexistence of a number of ethnic groups with different cultures in the same region can be studied from a variety of perspectives. This study focuses on the way each of these groups, with its own values, traditions and beliefs, has treated a category of deviants usually termed crazy, insane or mentally ill. To help the reader understand some of the dynamics at work, we will begin with a brief review of some elements of the history and political development of the region.

1.1 CONTROL OF THE REGION

This study deals with three ethnic groups*, the Loyalists, the Irish and the Acadians, who have lived together for more than two hundred years in the region that was once known as Acadia and is now called New Brunswick.

The geography of the region is as rich as its history. Its fertile plains, its rivers teeming with fish, its bays (Chaleurs and Fundy) and its vast and varied forests made it an ideal habitat for its native population, North American Indians of the Micmac and Maliseet tribes.

As time passed, European explorers, following in the footsteps of Christopher Columbus and Jacques Cartier, "discovered" the region. After the "discovery," a new stage in the region's history began, in which

---

* The term "ethnic groups" is used here in its broadest sense as a convenient designation for the three groups under study.

possession of territory and commercial interests were the dominant forces. At the time, New Brunswick was part of a colony called Arcadia, which also included Nova Scotia and Prince Edward Island. From the beginning, England, France and the New England colonies all wanted the territory, and this rivalry led to a number of armed conflicts. All three powers sought the right to fish, hunt and trade with the native people, as well as economic and political domination in the region.

The wars between France and England in the seventeenth and eighteenth centuries also affected Acadia. The region was attacked seven times in less than a century — in 1613, 1654, 1690, twice in 1704, again in 1707, and finally in 1710; on this last occasion, it fell into English hands for good, and France formally ceded it to England three years later. This period culminated in the infamous deportation of the Acadians in 1755, on the pretext that they refused to swear an oath of allegiance to the king of England. From 7,000 to 8,000 Acadians, who had wanted to remain neutral in the conflict between the two great powers, were deported between 1755 and 1762 on the orders of Governor Charles Lawrence. Today, scattered communities of Acadians can be found in both North America and Europe — in Louisiana, the Gaspé peninsula, St. Pierre and Miquelon, Spain, France. Meanwhile, about 5,000 Acadians fled into the woods and later settled in uninhabited parts of northwestern and southeastern New Brunswick, as well as at the northeastern and southwestern tips of Nova Scotia and in Prince Edward Island.

This was clearly exclusion for political reasons. In Europe during this period people banished the mad and the insane to get them out of the way. In Acadia, the authorities got rid of an entire people when it refused to submit.

A number of deportees returned to Acadia, which prompted Antonine Maillet to say: *And that's why, when Acadie wrenched itself out of exile at the end of the eighteenth century, it quit its crib so quiet, with never a wail nor a shout, without even clapping its hands. It came home by the back door, and on tiptoe. And when the world got round to noticing, it was too late; Acadie already had springs in its shanks and its nose in the wind.*[2]

The Acadians paid a high price for wanting to remain neutral and refusing to take sides in the conflict. They were contemptuously called "French Neutrals" because they did not want to side with the dominant English against their "mother country," France.

Working through their local agents, the English residents, the New England colonies were in a good position to dominate trade and development in the region. After Quebec fell into English hands in 1759, they gradually established an economic and political system in which Acadians and French-Canadians could choose only to forget or to submit.

1.2 REPOPULATION OF THE REGION

The governor of the time did not want to see New Brunswick's land remain idle, and so he invited people to move there from New England. Some 7,000 of them accepted the invitation, leaving their homes to move onto the land that had been untended since the Acadians "left." They came especially to the Bay of Fundy area, and the new inhabitants took charge of the political and economic life of the region. Other large waves of immigration followed, bringing primarily Loyalists and Irish to New Brunswick.

1.2.1 The Arrival of the Loyalists

The American Revolution had a major influence on the history of New Brunswick. When independence came, those Americans who had wanted the colonies to remain in English hands found themselves in a precarious position. With the leaders of the war of independence now in power, most of the Loyalists, as they were called, had to pack their bags and move north. The English authorities rewarded them for their loyalty by granting them land concessions, tools and supplies. They were given more than a million acres of free land in Canada. Twelve thousand Loyalists settled in New Brunswick, and their arrival had a considerable impact on the development of the region. Through Loyalist influence, the territory became a province in 1784, governed from Saint John by Lieutenant-Governor Thomas Carleton. The new provincial capital, Fredericton, was founded about this time. The motto chosen for the new province, *Spem Reduxit* (Hope is Reborn), reflected the feeling of the newly arrived Loyalists rather than that of the deported Acadians.

1.2.2 Irish Immigration

Many Irish were forced to leave their country because of famine, an unstable political situation, and a bleak future. In the early nineteenth century, some of them chose Canada as their new home. Most of those who came to New Brunswick became farmers, while others became merchants.

The region's population, which stood at 25,000 in 1803, mushroomed to 74,000 in 1824 and 193,000 in 1851. Immigration is clearly of crucial importance in New Brunswick's history, marked as it is by the large influx of Irish and Loyalists, along with Scottish and Dutch settlers.

In this brief historical outline, three ethnic groups which differ markedly from one another in their way of life, their religion, and their relation to economic and political power have been introduced.

1.3 CHARACTERISTICS OF THE THREE GROUPS UNDER STUDY

1.3.1 The Loyalists

From the time of their arrival, the Loyalists enjoyed the moral, financial and political support of the ruling colonial elite. They were able to manipulate conditions to their own advantage, and monopolize trade, seaports, the lumber industry, and the export of the products they purchased from the natives, the Acadians and the Irish. Through their efforts, the province's first higher education institution, the University of New Brunswick, was founded in 1829. It was purchased by the government thirty years later.

The Loyalists were a proud people, and they demanded special status so that they would never again have to face the kind of persecution they had suffered in the United States. They believed that their loyalty to England during the American Revolution placed them in a category above their fellow citizens, and they were encouraged in this belief. They quickly took control of the region, establishing economic and political structures suited to their needs and actively participating in the process of industrialization that was then just getting underway in North America. Being in an English colony, the Loyalists insisted on being honoured just as those who had fought against England were in the United States. Defeated in a war in which their privileged class interests were opposed to those of the majority, they tried to regain their superior social status in Canada.

Here is how one New Brunswicker of Loyalist stock, interviewed for this study, views what happened:

The difference between the two [the Loyalists and the Acadians] was that we were an educated group of people … We brought education with us when we came … The Loyalists brought their culture with them; the French were more backward … It took courage for us to leave our homes and come to a place we didn't know … When we came here and to Nova

Scotia, we brought a form of government with us too.

The literature tells us that even in the eighteenth century, the Loyalists lived very well. According to one account, they had "bread, butter and cheese in abundance. In many instances, you may discover not only the comforts of life, but luxuries procured by their over-plus produce. ... Their barns contain a stock of cattle, horses, sheep and swine, of more value than their ancestors in New Jersey or New England possessed."[3]

It is well known that in the United States these people had refused to support the emergence of an independent government standing for equality, democracy and freedom. It could be expected that, when they were in a position of power, they would try to prevent the establishment of such a government.

With their business acumen, they were able to control markets, trade and industrial development and keep political power in their own hands.

1.3.2 The Irish

Irish immigration to New Brunswick took place primarily as a result of the Irish rebellion of 1798 and the famine of 1822. The Irish continued in the rural way of life they had known in their homeland. They currently make up 15 per cent of the population of the Atlantic region. Since most of them were Catholics, it would be expected that they would feel an affinity with the Acadians. But history tells us that, on the contrary, the two groups clashed over language; the Irish were interested in obtaining power and in establishing an English-speaking religious hierarchy throughout eastern Canada. One manifestation of this clash was the Acadians' struggle to secure the appointment of an Acadian bishop. It took more than twenty-five years of effort and several trips to Rome by Acadian representatives before the question was finally resolved in 1913. By this time, English-speaking Catholics — most of whom were Irish — already had five bishops in the Atlantic region.

Until the twentieth century, the church hierarchy was opposed to the use of French in the church in Acadia, believing that English, the language of the majority, would be a better vehicle to spread Catholicism in Canada. Unilingual English-speaking priests were often named to French parishes to promote the use of English in religious ceremonies. In addition, the Collège St-Louis in St-Louis de Kent, the most important educational institution serving the Acadian population, was closed in 1882 because the bishop of Chatham, who provided the funds for the school, believed that the use of French was being unduly encouraged.

As Anglophones, the Irish were accepted fairly easily by the ruling elite of the province. With their business and organizational skills, their interests were well represented at the various levels of political and economic power. The financial and political prestige of the Irish in the Acadian regions and the difference in status between them and the Acadians were especially striking. In many an Acadian village at that time, the provincial government was represented by an Anglophone who carried out a variety of administrative duties. The government chose a representative who could communicate in English with provincial authorities, and at the same time be accepted by the local Acadian population by virtue of his Catholic faith.

Anglophones exerted local control and had considerable political power throughout the region, even in the smallest communities. When Acadians wanted things done, they had to deal either with this political bloc or with the religious hierarchy, also under English control.

1.3.3 The Acadians

Being in a minority position, the Acadians have tended to try to get along with everyone and have been encouraged by their church authorities to be passive. Nevertheless, they have always had to fight for recognition and for their rights. As Michel Roy has written:

At one point, the Acadians suffered brutal violence: the deportation. Since then, they have fought stubbornly and relentlessly against another kind of violence, aimed at keeping them in a state of almost total subordination. Up to that point, they battled constantly for the basic right to live. Afterwards, they exhausted themselves in endless struggles for property rights, political rights, educational rights, language rights — not to mention the question of economic status.[4]

According to the 1981 census, 36.1 per cent of the population of New Brunswick is of French ethnic origin. The Parti Acadien has represented the political interests of progressive Acadians. Its platform included a call for a separate Acadian geographic entity which would have meant dividing the province as it now stands in two. The party received 3,331 votes in the 1982 provincial election. It did not run any candidates in the 1987 election.

On the basis of per capita income, Acadians can be considered disadvantaged relative to the Anglophone population. Edmund Aunger of the University of Alberta has compared the political and economic

Table 1
Income Stratification in New Brunswick (1971)

Annual income, $	% of English	% of French	% of Total
5,000+	25	17	22
3,000 - 4,999	15	13	14
1,000 - 2,999	22	25	23
0 - 999	39	44	41
Total	101	99	100
Number	288,515	142,980	431,495

Source: Edmund Aunger, *In Search of Political Stability* (Montreal: McGill-Queen's, 1981), p. 97.

development of New Brunswick Acadians with that of Catholics in Northern Ireland. Table 1, taken from his study, shows the disparities between Anglophones and Francophones in New Brunswick. The table demonstrates that on the average, Anglophones have a higher annual income than Francophones. There is a similar disparity in the educational levels of the two groups, as shown in table 2. Thus, in both income and education, there is a significant difference between the two language groups, and in both cases it is the Acadians who are disadvantaged.

Aunger concludes that the accommodationist strategy of *bon-ententisme,* which the Acadian elite and clergy advocate so strongly, is an essential element in preserving the political status quo in Acadian-Anglophone relations and helps maintain Anglophone domination as the basis of the social order in Acadia. Aunger argues that the *bon-ententisme* of the Acadian elite, as opposed to the more uncompromising, militant stand taken by the Catholic elite of Northern Ireland, is the major reason New Brunswick Acadians passively accept inequality while the minority in Northern Ireland is in revolt.

Michel Roy's thesis is that the Acadians' Catholicism has worked against political and economic emancipation. In espousing a form of nationalism that preached cooperation instead of confrontation, the elite successfully conveyed the idea that power is not of this world, and thus contributed to the alienation and assimilation of the Acadians.

Table 2
Educational Stratification in New Brunswick (1971)

Years of schooling	% of English	% of French	% of Total
13+	9	6	8
9 - 12	52	30	45
5 - 8	34	44	37
0 - 5	5	20	10
Total	100	100	100
Number	246,645	120,230	366,875

Source: Edmund Aunger, *In Search of Political Stability* (Montreal: McGill-Queen's, 1981), p. 95.

In fact, the continued existence of the Acadian minority is a result of its quiet acceptance of its lot. To a large degree, Acadians depend on the mercy of the dominant ethnic group for their collective survival. "French Acadians, your respect for the law and your religious devotion are a bulwark for our country against the revolutionary invasion of socialism," said a Nova Scotia politician early in the century.[5]

And yet, Nova Scotia has an assimilation rate of 32.1 per cent (1981). In Acadia as elsewhere, the English language is an unparalleled instrument of domination. According to Bernard Cassen:

Language issues cannot be viewed as merely technical questions. To do so is to acquiesce in the classic tactic of dominant groups, who always find rational, economic arguments to legitimize their superior position. ... Some local elites not only took it for granted that the language of business or technology was English but themselves insisted on gaining access to knowledge of the language as a sign that they belonged to the world of power. English thus became one of the ways of excluding the less privileged. The use of English became an indicator of class, or at least a "status symbol" for upper management. It sealed the alliance of "for-ward-looking" local bourgeoisies with American interests.[6]

The history of the three groups shows unequal development, differing needs, and almost diametrically opposed aspirations. These differences are rooted in religious beliefs: in the case of the Loyalists, these beliefs encouraged the accumulation of wealth, while in the case of the Acadians and the Irish, they encouraged passivity, modesty and humility. Passivity, in both religious and civil life, was a basic tenet of the Acadian value structure.⟩

The Protestant ethic did not simply accept the idea of wealth: it made the accumulation of wealth a duty. All respectable citizens were expected to put their property to productive use, spend carefully, and reinvest their profits in order to generate more capital. The successful person was considered honourable, success being regarded as almost divinely ordained. As John Kenneth Galbraith put it, "once again, religion went hand in hand with real property conveyancing, somewhat disguising the role of the latter. ... For Puritans and Protestants spiritual merit lay with the homestead and family farm."[7] The rise of the Loyalist communities and other White Anglo-Saxon Protestants is quite understandable when considered in this light.

The Acadians inherited a very different religious ethic, based mainly on submissiveness, poverty and respect for authority, as if these were signs of obedience to God's will. The established order and all authority, even civil authority, were sanctioned by religion and considered divine.

These different peoples lived side by side in a region that belonged to and was run by England. With their enterprising spirit and the business sense imparted to them by their religion, the Loyalists were imbued with a moral code, a way of organizing their lives and an ability to look to the future. This was concretized in the social system they created, based on private enterprise and the perception of economic and political power as a sign of God's blessing.

The Irish, for their part, were an interesting group by virtue of their position between the language-religion poles represented by the other two groups. As Anglophones, they were able to gain a measure of power, while as Catholics, they played a part in the domination of the Acadians in the religious sphere.

Table 3 shows that in 1871, the rate of illiteracy was up to ten times higher in counties with large Francophone concentrations than in majority Anglophone counties. This table points to the rather dismal situation of the Acadians in the last century. They had few schools and no funds either to set up a school system or to pay competent teachers. Louis J. Robichaud relates that even in 1960, when he was premier of New Brunswick, one country school had 125 pupils in all eight elementary grades in a single room. The teacher was simply a student who had failed her eighth grade

Table 3
Illiteracy and Education Rates for the Counties of New Brunswick and the Four Founding Provinces of Canada (1871)

County	French Ethnic Origin (% of County)	Illiteracy[1] (% of population)	Education[2] (% of population)
Albert	0.7	16	40
Carleton	2.0	8	42
Charlotte	0.8	9	48
Gloucester	67.0	53	19
Kent	56.0	49	23
Kings	1.0	10	31
Northumberland	6.0	21	41
Queens	0.9	8	40
Restigouche	19.0	17	23
St. John	0.6	14	46
Saint John (city)	0.6	13	51
Sunbury	2.0	17	35
Victoria[3]	61.0	53	18
Westmorland	31.0	30	34
York	2.0	11	35
New Brunswick	15	21	36
Nova Scotia	n.a.	25	57
Quebec	n.a.	45	41
Ontario	n.a.	13	61
Total (four provinces)	n.a.	26	52

1. 20 years old and over
2. 5 to 20 years old
3. Includes Madawaska county (the two counties were separated in 1873).

Source : Canada, Department of Agriculture, *Census of Canada 1871*, volume 7, table 3; volume 2, table 10.

at the same school the year before.[8]

The report of the New Brunswick Royal Commission on Finance and Municipal Taxation (1963) set up by Premier Robichaud criticized such flagrant injustices as the fact that in the Acadian county of Kent $132 was allocated per student, while in the Anglophone county of Sunbury the figure was $331. The cycle of poverty was firmly implanted in the Acadian areas; per capita income was six times higher in Sunbury than in Kent. It should therefore come as no surprise that 26 per cent of the patients admitted to the Restigouche Hospital Center between 1979 and 1982 were functionally illiterate, and that people from the Acadian Peninsula were eight times more likely to have educational difficulties than other New Brunswickers.

Since the Deportation, the Loyalists have created a secure place for themselves in, business and the professions, while the unknown and neglected Acadians have had to get along with marginal jobs in a subsistence economy. During the 1970s, despite a massive equal opportunity program, Acadians still worked primarily in the resource sector and in manufacturing. High technology, modern industrial, specialized and management jobs were occupied by Anglophones. Figure 1 illustrates these differences: the higher a job's social status, the more likely it is to be held by an Anglophone. Francophones hold jobs at the lower end of the economic and occupational scale, which require less training and are less remunerative. They are caught in a vicious circle.

The two maps in figure 2 (page 27) illustrate this phenomenon by looking at families receiving financial assistance from the government in the 1970s — a time when the Equal Opportunity program was in full operation. The first map shows the percentage of Francophone residents in various parts of the province, while the second gives a regional breakdown of the rate of social assistance in the province in 1972-73. When the two maps are compared, they show that:

• the Francophone population is concentrated in the northwest, northeast and southeast parts of the province;
• the percentage of welfare recipients is significantly higher in these areas;
• dependence on social assistance is greater in the Acadian Peninsula (in the northeast part of the province) than in any other region;
• the southern part of the province has a lower rate of social assistance, indicating that this area is more highly developed economically.

How has the situation changed in the 1980s?

A recent study comparing various regions of the province shows that

Figure 1
Occupational Categories by Language
Group, New Brunswick, 1968

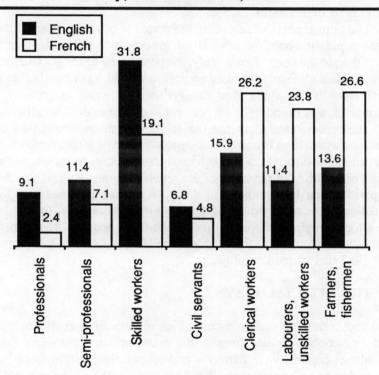

Source: Alain Even, "Le Territoire pilote du Nouveau-Brunswick ou les blocages culturels au développement économique", doctoral thesis, Faculté de droit et de sciences économiques, Université de Rennes, 1970, p. 314.

Note: In the original table the total did not add to 100 per cent for the French categories.

in 1981 the per capita gross domestic product of the Acadian regions was only 83.7 per cent of that of the province as a whole, and 56.4 per cent of the Canadian figure. At the same time, unemployment was 62 per cent higher in northern New Brunswick than in the south. In addition, a member of the province's work force had to provide for the needs of 0.83 individuals outside the work force in the north, as compared with only 0.68 individuals in the south.

The same report indicates that, in the area of education, the percentage of the population holding university degrees was 51 per cent higher in the south than in the north. Conversely, the percentage of the population with no more than elementary school education was 41.5 per cent higher in the north than in the south. And finally, the death rate in northern New Brunswick was found to be 16 per cent higher than the Canadian figure.

The report concluded that the regions in the northern part of the province with a high Francophone concentration — 80 per cent or over — were the most disadvantaged both in overall socio-economic terms and in terms of health.[9] On the basis of the report's figures we can say that the disparities that have existed in the past are not disappearing. Recent statistics on the confinement of Acadians in psychiatric institutions show the effect of regional disparity on disadvantaged people: 78 per cent of the individuals admitted to the Restigouche Hospital Center between 1979 and 1982 had no paid employment.

1.4 THE OFFICIAL VIEW

The above analysis stands in contradiction to the way both Anglophone and Francophone elites present the situation. In their view the two founding peoples live in harmony and cooperation. Anglophone leaders go so far as to congratulate the Acadians on their tenacity and their willingness to accept an inferior status:

After the creation of the Province of New Brunswick in 1784 the Acadians were given grants of land and treated as British subjects. The Acadians were not "absorbed" by the English who came later to settle the region. They retained their French language, religion and culture. Nowhere is there to be found a group of people more aware of their history. Today Acadians account for about 35% of the total population of the province and play a very active part in every aspect of New Brunswick political, economic and social life.[10]

The Francophone elite also boasts about this spirit of cooperation which has been used to keep Acadians in an inferior position: *Indeed, we*

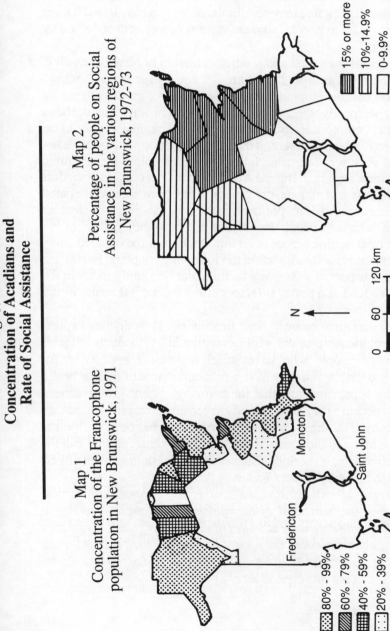

Concentration of Acadians and
Rate of Social Assistance

Map 1
Concentration of the Francophone
population in New Brunswick, 1971

Fredericton

Moncton

Saint John

80% - 99%
60% - 79%
40% - 59%
20% - 39%

Source: Statistics Canada, 1971.

Map 2
Percentage of people on Social
Assistance in the various regions of
New Brunswick, 1972-73

15% or more
10% - 14.9%
0 - 9.9%

Source: Jean-Claude Vernex, *Les francophones du Nouveau-Brunswick*,
thesis, Université de Lyon II, 1975, p. 571.

0   60   120 km

N

in New Brunswick exemplify the mutual tolerance and understanding that could well be emulated more fully in some of our sister provinces, in any bi-cultural nation.[11]

Both elites uphold a conciliatory line aimed at maintaining the current unequal situation. This game may benefit the elites that play it, but it does no good for the Acadian people, who are victims of a system endorsed by their own leaders.

In our sketch of the social and political situation in New Brunswick, we saw that the three groups studied are not equal in terms of political power and economic development. Moreover, the three groups see reality from different perspectives, based on their different histories, which have given them different conceptions of sociopolitical reality. It should be noted that, even for the Loyalists and the Irish, economic development has lagged behind what was occurring in industrial and commercial centres elsewhere in North America. But the Acadians have not only been victims of regional disparity and national oppression. They have been so alienated historically, economically and politically that they can be considered an oppressed and colonized people (see figure 3, pp. 29-30).

This historical outline serves as an introduction to the detailed study of mental health in New Brunswick in the following chapters. Social and political history is part of a people's culture, and this study looks at the ways in which social and political factors affect the mental health of the three groups.

Can Acadians feel at home in New Brunswick? How do they express their cultural relationship to the world they live in? What is the state of mental health of people who have suffered national oppression for centuries? Is it possible that they have a particular view of mental health because of this oppression, and that the two Anglophone groups have a different view because they are more privileged and better integrated into industrial society? Has the Acadians' history, which has been difficult in so many ways, affected their mental health? In this sense, can we call the Acadian situation a "calm period of successful colonisation," with effects similar to those noted by Frantz Fanon in Africa?

In the period of colonisation when it is not contested by armed resistance, when the sum total of harmful nervous stimuli overstep a certain threshold, the defensive attitudes of the natives give way and they then find themselves crowding the mental hospitals. There is thus during this calm period of successful colonisation a regular and important mental pathology which is the direct product of oppression.[12]

Figure 3
Comparison of the Three Groups Studied

Point of Comparison	Acadians	Irish	Loyalists
Political situation	Oppressed minority, dependent	Minority with some power because of language	Colonizing majority integrated into North American society
Consequences of inequality	Self-denigration, self-colonization	Survival, economic and political integration	Development of networks, integration of resources through exports and urbanization
Type of economy	Subsistence: fishing, agriculture, industrial labour	Markets better organized, some industrial ventures	Control of business and industry, control of trans-portation routes (seaports,etc.)
Areas of influence of elites	Clerical elite	Industrial and clerical elite	Industrial and political elite
Political role	Lower-level civil servants	Better organized politically	Control of political life
First language	French	English	English
Second language	English	None	None
Language of work	English	English	English

	Catholic	Catholic	Protestant
Religion	Catholic	Catholic	Protestant
Educational level	First generation of university students	Second and third generations of university students	Third and fourth generations of university students
Main occupations	Technical, resource industry	Resource and secondary industry, business	Management, administration, professional
Important historical factors	Deportation; Equal Opportunity program, 1967	Immigration policies	American independence, land concessions and other benefits
Number of members elected to the Legislative Assembly between 1900 and 1958	14/79	10/79 (English Catholic members)	55/79 (English Protestant members)
Distance from centres of decision-making	Distant, marginal	Close, peripheral	Central
Instruments of economic control	Life insurance, credit unions	Markets, farms, internal trade	Cities, seaports, foreign trade, communications, oil
Attitude	Acceptance of history, change and development through cooperation	Alliance with economic power, religious control	Conquest and control of the region and resources
Trends	Emigration, assimilation	Association with cooperation	Domination through dominant majority

NOTES

1. Quoted by Thomas Szasz, *The Theology of Medicine* (Baton Rouge: Louisiana State University Press, 1977), p. 6.
2. Antonine Maillet, *Pelagie* (Garden City, N.Y.: Doubleday, 1982), p. 1.
3. Chester Martin, "The Loyalists in New Brunswick," *Ontario Historical Society* 30 (1934): 165 - 66.
4. Michel Roy, *L'Acadie perdue* (Montreal: Québec/Amérique, 1978), pp. 24 -25.
5. Ibid., p. 129.
6. Bernard Cassen, "La langue anglaise comme véhicule de l'impérialisme culturel," *L'homme et la société,* nos. 47-50 (Jan.-Déc. 1978), pp. 95, 97.
7. John Kenneth Galbraith, *The New Industrial State* (London: Andre Deutsch, 1972), p. 51.
8. Information taken from *Le Programme Chance égale pour tous* ; a tape produced by the Ecole de Service Social of the Université de Moncton, November 1981.
9. See Jean-Bernard Robichaud, *La santé des francophones* , 3 vols. (Moncton: Editions d'Acadie, 1985), 1:139 -159.
10. Robert Fellow, *Researching Your Ancestors in New Brunswick* (Fredericton, n.d.), p. 11.
11. Louis Robichaud, "The Acadian Outlook (1)," in *French Canada Today*, edited by C.F. MacRae (Sackville, N.B.: Mount Allison University, 1961), p. 25.
12. Frantz Fanon, *The Wretched of the Earth* (New York: Grove Press, 1966), p. 204.

2

History of the Institutions

*Confinement is determined less
by mental illness than by the
vagaries of life.*
— Erving Goffman

*Mrs. Z., aged 72, admitted for
the twenty-second time for her
routine electroshock treatment.*
— a case history

2.1 THE CONFINEMENT OF DEVIANTS IN PSYCHIATRIC INSTITUTIONS

We all hope under the wise leadership of Doctor R. A. Gregory that the Provincial Hospital will operate as a ship carrying a heavy burden or load of precious lives', and steer to the course of tranquillity and prosperity. For the unfortunate class of our beloved citizens and with determination as our aim for their recoveries respectively, the ship will "Sail on." [1]

These words praising the director of the first psychiatric institution in the province (and in Canada) were spoken at the institution's 140th anniversary celebration in 1967. The passage contains the words *sail, ship* and *tranquillity.* These same terms were used in writings of the sixteenth and seventeenth centuries, the period when the institutional history of mental illness in the West began. Michel Foucault explores the use of these images:

Frequently [in the Middle Ages] they were handed over to boatmen ... Often the cities of Europe must have seen these "ships of fools" approaching their harbours ... It is for the other world that the madman sets sail in his fool's boat; it is from the other world that he comes when he disembarks. Confined on the ship, from which there is no escape, the madman is delivered to the river with its thousand arms, the sea with its thousand roads, to that great uncertainty external to everything. He is a prisoner in the midst of what is the freest, the openest of routes. [2]

This chapter looks at mental illness both from the perspective of institutional and legal history and from the perspective of the victims of this modern-day form of leprosy. It should be noted that in New Brunswick psychiatric facilities and institutions developed in Saint John, industrial capital of the province, bustling seaport and quintessential Loyalist city.

2.1.1 Early Legislation and Institutions

New Brunswick legislation dealing with indigents and their treatment followed the English model. From the time of colonization, the famous Poor Law implemented under Elizabeth I in 1601 was in force in New Brunswick; accordingly, the poor were the responsibility of the parish where they were born or where they were domiciled. In economically favoured areas, unemployment was rare and the law could be implemented without serious financial consequences. Only a very small portion of the budget was required for the few poor people who could find no place in the labour market. In poorer regions, however, cities, villages and counties devoted the lion's share of their budgets to fulfilling their responsibility to care for indigents. This was the case in the Francophone counties of New Brunswick.

In 1786, New Brunswick passed its own Poor Law. It was based on New England legislation, which was in turn copied from the mother country's Poor Law. Each county was given full responsibility for its own indigents, including old people, abandoned children, mad people, and criminals, all of whom were to be treated in the same way. The more fortunate counties had workhouses where all these people were sent. The rest tried to place them in special homes; otherwise, they were sent to prison, and mad people, who were considered dangerous, were confined.

In 1824, New Brunswick passed a law applying specifically to the mentally ill. It authorized "any two Justices of the Peace to issue a warrant for the apprehension of a lunatic or mad person, and cause him to be kept safely locked in some secure place directed and appointed by them, and, if they deemed it to be necessary, to be chained."[3]

In New Brunswick as elsewhere, laws and institutions went together. Under the provisions of the 1824 legislation, the mentally disturbed, insane and demented could be shut away and chained. But prisons were not the answer, so parliament approved a request by municipal authorities for permission to establish an asylum.

Irish immigrants brought a serious cholera epidemic when they landed in Saint John in 1832, and a building had to be found to quarantine them. When the epidemic was over, the authorities decided to use the building as a permanent facility to house and care for another category of social outcasts, mad people. And when the new facility opened its doors in 1836, it was called the Provincial Lunatic Asylum, a name it kept until 1903.

Thus, once madness was explicitly identified and named, it was organized. In France, the industrial city of Lyon boasted of having opened its psychiatric institution thirty years before Paris, the national capital. Similarly, the flourishing industrial centre of Saint John could claim to have the first institution in New Brunswick and even in Canada. But it would only be in 1954, 118 years later, that a second institution of this kind would be opened, in Campbellton in the northeastern part of the province.

2.1.2 The Inmates

Who was sent to the psychiatric institution in the nineteenth century? An investigation of case histories dated between 1875 and 1899 reveals that people were committed for all kinds of reasons, including intemperance, jealousy, poverty, malaria, dental problems, loneliness, masturbation, and tobacco use. The situation was remarkably similar to that in Europe where, as Foucault noted, "in a hundred and fifty years, confinement had become the abusive amalgam of heterogeneous elements."[4]

Georges Devereux formulated the criticism in another way: how is it possible to determine who is mentally ill if psychiatry has no definition of mental illness? "Whereas anthropologists write a great deal about their key concept," Devereux wrote, "the problem of what is 'normal' and what is 'abnormal' has received relatively little systematic attention in recent psychiatric literature."[5]

From the beginning, the authorities were faced with serious problems. Some patients did not fit the goals of the institution, and it was not easy to define the term "insane and demented." In 1858 the first superintendent of the asylum, Dr. Waddell, had this to say on the subject: "Were the arrangements for the parish poor ... all they ought to be and the laws so amended that the harmless, imbecile and the delirious might be excluded from this establishment, then our tables of mortality would exhibit a correct percentage on insanity."[6]

This passage indicates that government authorities and people in general were taking advantage of the new institution, sending individuals to it who in one way or another did not fit into the existing social structure of the time. As Roger Gentis put it, "more and more, the unwanted — the retarded, the old, the alcoholic, and soon, perhaps, the deformed and the lame — are put away, banished, got rid of."[7]

During that period, the care varied according to the victim's social class and proximity to the services offered. The most fortunate were able to go outside the province to Europe or the United States to receive what was considered higher-quality treatment. People who lived in Saint John and the surrounding area could go to the Provincial Lunatic Asylum. For those to whom these options were closed because of language, money or distance, the only recourse was the Poor Law. They had to remain at home or else enter one of the county homes.

It was understood that the patient's parish of residence had financial responsibility in such cases. Thus, as recently as the early twentieth century, the poor, helpless and mad were auctioned off. Buyers acquired these unfortunates to extract as much work as possible from them, whether on the farm, in the fisheries, in gardens and homes, or elsewhere. In her novel *Les Cordes de Bois*, Antonine Maillet relates that auctions continued to take place up until the 1930s, especially in the Acadian villages in Kent County.

Judging by the first annual report of the Provincial Lunatic Asylum, people quickly learned to use the new institution for the "insane and demented." Thirty-one individuals were admitted in the first year. Of those, six were released "cured," five were released "improved," two were released with "no improvement," and four died.* Fourteen remained in the institution at the end of the first year, of whom eleven showed "no visible improvement."

Having studied the first annual report, Dr. Dorothy Chen has this to say:

In studying the accounts — it is remarkable that actual expenses are recorded only for the keeping of patients and the purchasing of straight jackets; but no allowance was made for the repairs and maintenance of the building and furniture ... Some of the details of the itemized accounts are highly suggestive of ... the methods of treatment, in which bloodletting must have played a considerable part.[8]

The institutional solution must have been a good one, judging by its popularity. Only three years after the first institution was opened, a committee was formed to select the site for a permanent institution with room for ninety patients. In 1848, the new institution, located just outside the city of Saint John, opened its doors.

Saint John held itself up as a model not only of industrial development but also of morality and normality. The principles of industrialization were applied to health, and in particular to mental health. A healthy person

---

* No study of deaths in psychiatric institutions in New Brunswick has yet been done. An *a priori* observation is that a remarkable number of people die in such institutions for more or less dubious reasons.

was someone who could work and contribute to building a "better society", a mad person was someone who did not adapt and could not fit in. As York University sociologist John O'Neill has written:

Thus colonial medicine and psychology diagnose the lives of the oppressed in abstraction from the political conditions of which they are themselves an integral practice. This diagnosis is fundamentally racist, as Fanon has shown, in the sense that the oppressors' language only serves to locate political differences racially.[9]

The ways in which people are oppressed by psychiatric institutions and their agents can be seen through a few examples. The following report concerns an eighteen-year-old woman from a Francophone area of the province, Mrs. X, admitted to the Saint John psychiatric hospital in 1966. The psychiatrist preparing the report did not speak French:

"I was not able to converse much with Mrs. X, because of the language barrier. Before she finished telling her story, she began to speak French, which I don't understand. No productive discussion took place." His diagnosis: schizophrenia.

In 1961, another psychiatrist at the same hospital entered the following report in the file of Mr. Y, a fifty-eight-year-old Acadian:

"This patient does not speak English very well. He usually sits still and does not speak. He is introverted and nothing interests him. He didn't even come to the birthday party that was organized for him." He diagnosed Mr. Y as psychotic. The third time he was institutionalized, Mr. Y remained in the hospital for six years. The following comment appears in his file: "a quiet man and very cooperative."

Obviously these psychiatrists did not take into account the language and culture of the members of an oppressed group or their alienation in an Anglophone psychiatric setting.

One professional recounts that in 1982 a patient used the term "*se fermer la boîte*" — a colloquial expression literally meaning "to shut one's box" and used in the same way as "to shut up" — in the course of discussing his problem with a psychiatrist. The doctor sent him to a psychiatric institution, indicating in his report that the individual was seriously disturbed and had hallucinations. According to the doctor, the individual wanted to "*s'enfermer dans une boîte*" — shut himself up in a box. Significantly, the doctor had just arrived in the country and had probably never heard the expression.

Who is confined to a psychiatric institution? A study of admissions from 1875 to 1899 shows that all kinds of people were admitted. However, proportions vary substantially with social status. In table 4, occupations

Table 4
Psychiatric Admissions by Occupation, New Brunswick, 1875-99

Occupation	% of Admissions
A. Daily workers and non-tradespersons	
1. Daily workers	16.7
2. Housewives	14.2
3. No occupation	10.7
4. House servants	7.6
B. Manual workers	
1. Farmers and wives	17.7
2. Milkmen, wives and daughters	.9
3. Seamen and wives	1.6
4. Merchants	1.6
C. Professionals	
1. Gentlemen	2.3
2. Teachers	1.4
3. Clergy	0.2
4. Physicians and wives	0.2

Table 5
Psychiatric Admissions by Occupation, New Brunswick, 1956-81

Occupation	No. of Admissions	% of Admissions	Cumulative %
No occupation	218	37.3	37.3
Housewives	133	22.7	60.0
Seasonal workers	85	14.5	74.5
Tradespersons (electricians, vendors, farmers, mechanics, etc.)	94	16.1	90.6
Students	23	3.9	94.5
Professionals	18	3.1	97.6
Unknown and other	14	2.4	100.0
Total	**585**	**100.0**	

are divided into three categories, and the four occupations with the highest percentages of admission are highlighted in each category. The table shows that unskilled labourers and people with no paid occupation were subject to confinement in psychiatric institutions more often than people in the other occupational categories.

For my doctoral dissertation, I studied 585 files of individuals admitted to the psychiatric hospitals in Saint John and Campbellton between 1956 and 1981 (see table 5). These files allow us to do an occupational comparison between people admitted during this period and those admitted in the nineteenth century. A few remarks can be made about these two tables:

• Both in the nineteenth century and now, the individuals most often admitted are people without work and people in occupations considered economically marginal, such as housewives and seasonal workers.

• While the occupational categories are not identical in the two tables, people without work and marginal workers represent a total of 49.2 per cent of admissions between 1875 and 1899, and 74.5 per cent of admissions between 1956 and 1981.

• In both periods, few professionals were treated in psychiatric institutions.

2.1.3 Reasons for Confinement

Table 6 shows the "diseases" from which individuals admitted for treatment suffered, based on the diagnoses of some of the 3,174 people admitted between 1875 and 1899. The figures are again drawn from the study mentioned earlier.

The field of psychiatry is vast, and the psychiatric institution served a variety of purposes — Foucault's "abusive amalgam of heterogeneous elements." How can such diagnoses as "disease nasal bone," "undue lactation" or "coup de soleil" (sunburn) be explained? How can the large number of people admitted with no diagnosis at all be justified?

Have the reasons for admission changed in this regard? The case histories of the 585 individuals admitted between 1956 and 1981 who are the subjects of this study show the following diagnoses, among others:

• Mr. X was sent to a psychiatric institution by a judge after breaking into a vending machine. He wanted something to eat.

• Mr. Y has been admitted eighteen times and still has not undergone a psychiatric evaluation.

• Mr. V, forty-nine years old, lives in a special home. The people in

Table 6
Some Reasons for Admission, New Brunswick, 1875-99*

Diagnosis	No. of men	No. of women
A. Physical causes		
Coup de soleil	15	3
Disease nasal bone	2	0
Defective nervous system	51	53
Undue lactation	-	8
Bite of dog	1	-
Climacteric	-	13
B. Sexual causes		
Onanism	69	5
Venereal	5	1
Unrestrained vicious habits	17	7
C. Spiritual causes		
Religious excitement	17	21
D. Work-related reasons		
Business problems	5	-
Overwork	11	9
Vagrancy	10	6
E. Other deviances		
Tobacco	9	-
Intemperance	191	18
Felonious	7	0
Jealousy	2	1
Not assigned	184	204

*Since these historical data were collected a number of years ago by someone else, I cannot analyse them according to culture, religion or ethnic group or in other ways that I would like. I want to express my sincere thanks to Stan Matheson for having provided me with the document on which this table is based.

charge of the home want to go on holiday and have him admitted for the time they will be away.

• "We have in our files a form signed by Mrs. X, who wants her mother admitted to a psychiatric institution on any pretext whatsoever."

• Miss X, sixteen years old, is seeing a young man of nineteen. Her foster parents disapprove and have her admitted to a psychiatric institution.

Clearly, straitjackets still exist. The psychiatric institution has served a wide variety of purposes, and as the preceding examples show, even in the twentieth century people are admitted for all kinds of questionable reasons.

Judging by the number of admissions, the confinement of deviants in psychiatric institutions in the nineteenth century was a great success. The authorities had to expand the Saint John asylum three times, and the problem of overcrowding reappeared soon after each expansion.

2.1.4 The Historical Background, 1880-1980

Several events that took place in the late nineteenth and early twentieth centuries are important to our study.

In 1884, the Criminal Insane Law was passed in New Brunswick. According to this legislation, any infraction committed by an idiot, an imbecile or an insane person did not constitute a crime and the person was not legally responsible. But the law also said that the person could be sent to an asylum indefinitely, "there to remain until he is restored to his right mind."

When a similar law had been passed in England, the authorities had simply released those to whom it applied. Today, such individuals are sent to psychiatric institutions for indefinite periods. The only person who can authorize their release is the lieutenant-governor of the province, who can reevaluate their cases every six months.

In 1903, the Provincial Lunatic Asylum changed its name to Provincial Hospital because the old name was "evil sounding and revolting ... It is a sore trial enough to be compelled to commit one's relatives or friends without being compelled to advertise the fact by addressing mail or other matter to them at a lunatic asylum... The word 'hospital' substituted for 'asylum'... would be more in keeping with the aims and objects of the institution."[10] The name change reflected the fact that the institution was slowly remodelling its practices along medical lines. Admission procedures showed the same tendency, notably in relation to the question of who had the power to commit someone. Sending people to psychiatric institutions had been the prerogative of justices of the peace, but in 1905, under the revised "lunatic law," this power was transferred to the medical profession.

Since then, someone who wants to have a person confined against his will has had to call on a doctor practising in the province. If the doctor agrees to the request for admission for psychiatric evaluation, the individual is automatically admitted to an institution for a period of thirty days.

In the late nineteenth century efforts were made to meet the needs of individuals for whom the institution was not the answer. As early as 1884 the institutional authorities were looking for different forms of treatment for such patients and recommended that one group of patients be transferred to cottages or a farm. A Dr. Steeves, superintendent at the time, saw boarding some patients outside the institution as a possibility and was active in trying to find solutions of that kind. In his annual report of 1892, he stated: "Whilst it is true that no system of redistributing insane persons among the people has met with substantial success, yet such attempts have not been abandoned."[11]

In 1891 Dr. Steeves had objected to criminals being placed in the hospital. He saw this practice as contrary to the purpose of the institution, as the presence of criminals would effectively turn the hospital into a prison with guards, locks and bars.

A century later there still appears to be no answer to the question of what kind of people should be admitted to psychiatric institutions. American studies have shown that 5 per cent of psychiatric patients are considered dangerous — the same proportion as in the population as a whole. Why then do people think of individuals held in psychiatric institutions as dangerous, and why is it so difficult to return anyone who has spent any time at all in such an institution to the community?

In 1980, a survey at the Centracare psychiatric hospital (formerly the Saint John psychiatric hospital) showed that in the view of the staff, more than 70 per cent of the patients had no reason to be there. If the personnel who handle the day-to-day care of the victims of an institution feel that more than two-thirds of them are there for no reason, whose purposes does the institution serve?

Thus, a psychiatric nursing aide observed that "after working here for five years, I often wonder who is sicker, the psychiatrists or the patients. The uniform is often the only way to tell them apart." What are we to make of such a statement? Perhaps it is just another way of saying what R.D. Laing wrote: "I think, however, that schizophrenics have more to teach psychiatrists about the inner world than psychiatrists their patients."[12]

Another aspect of the institution is evoked by Mr. X, eighteen years old and admitted in 1971: "If I stay here any longer, I'll go crazy for sure."

In 1942 and 1943, an electroshock therapy clinic was set up at the Saint John psychiatric hospital. A woman who worked there described it in the following terms:

Most patients were tied down, either by the arms or by the ankles. We put straitjackets on the most agitated ones. When we took a straitjacket off, the patient's skin was raw and bleeding because he had worn it so long. Often bits of flesh were stuck to it. The most violent ones were put in individual cages where they could only stick their fingers out. They only had some straw for a mattress, and we changed it when it got too dirty and full of excrement.

A social worker confirmed that cages were still in everyday use in the 1960s.

Although the hospital was expanded several times, it regularly suffered from overcrowding. In 1948, for example, it officially had 850 beds, but there were more than 1,400 patients. With a second psychiatric institution in Campbellton (in the northern part of the province) not yet open, the number went as high as 1,701 in 1953. Of these, 350 lived in a rat-infested firetrap called the Annex.

2.1.5 Treatment

It is difficult to judge the forms of treatment used in these institutions, or even to know what they were. Annual reports that deal with the subject and provide figures indicate that the preferred treatment was either insulin or electroconvulsive (commonly known as electroshock) therapy. Table 7 (p. 46) summarizes the research on this question.

Insulin-shock treatment was first mentioned in 1933 by a Dr. Sakel. Apparently, good results were obtained, particularly in the treatment of schizophrenia. Deep-insulin treatment was still used in the 1950s, while the use of modified-insulin treatment continued into the 1960s. Electroconvulsive therapy was in use for a longer period and, as of 1983, was still a common treatment at Centracare, according to its director. However, statistics on the frequency of its use have not been published since 1968.

Electroshock therapy was used with more women (1,943) than men (1,340). Insulin-shock treatment was used more often with men than with women, but the difference was less marked — 526 to 465. The following quotations from case histories of the 1960s and 1970s show the effects of some of the methods of treatment that were used:

• Mrs. X, twenty-three years old. The psychiatrist notes that "this patient suffers from mental confusion, perhaps caused by her many electroconvulsive therapy sessions" (1966).

• Mrs. Z, seventy-seven years old. Admitted twenty-two times. "Mrs. Z has come for her routine electroshock. She has been depressed for the last fifty years."

• Mrs. V, forty-one years old. Admitted for the fifth time in 1981. During her first period of hospitalization, which lasted fourteen years, she was treated with electroshock, deep coma, Stelazine, Tofranil, Mellaril and Surmontil. She has now come to the hospital in a catatonic state.

• Mrs. M, fifty-eight years old. Admitted in 1961. It is recorded in her file that she said: "I was locked up in a closet 60 cm by 120 cm and given a blanket. It was the middle of winter; there was no heating and it was very cold. A thirty-five-year-old woman had died there not long before."

From table 7 and the preceding statements, it can be seen that methods of treatment for the mentally ill used at any given time are related to other developments taking place in society at the same time. Insulin was discovered in 1920 and given to the mentally ill beginning in 1932. In the same way, electrical energy was put to use in the treatment of the mentally ill beginning in the 1940s. In the 1960s, these treatments were replaced by drugs, which are now hailed as a miracle cure. Many "treatments" in the past — including cold showers, lobotomy and bloodletting — were similarly hailed.

2.1.6 Other Institutions

In addition to the two institutions in Saint John and Campbellton, institutional psychiatric services in the early 1980s included the William F. Roberts Hospital School, a hospital for children (closed in 1985); and the Riverglade Memorial Hospital, a geriatric hospital which was formerly a tuberculosis treatment centre and now specializes in psychiatric services for senior citizens.

The two psychiatric institutions changed their administrative structures in 1980, each acquiring a board of directors. They also both changed their names: the Saint John psychiatric hospital to Centracare and the Campbellton institution to Restigouche Hospital Center.

We can see that New Brunswick was no different from Europe and the rest of North America in adopting the institutional model. In some ways, the province was ahead of other areas in this respect. The first institution

Table 7
Forms of Treatment, New Brunswick, 1954-68

Year	Sex	Deep-Insulin Treatment		Modified-Insulin Treatment		Electroconvulsive Therapy	
		Patients Treated	Sessions	Patients Treated	Sessions	Patients Treated	Sessions
1954	M	7	-	31	-	68	1207
	F	21	-	15	-	85	1113
1955	M	12	677	53	1077	92	1535
	F	18	508	51	1254	142	1958
1956	M	16	647	80	1866	127	1239
	F	11	318	67	1207	195	1492
1957-58	M	13	691	92	1841	130	1439
	F	9	285	48	967	160	1883
1958-59	M	23	401	84	1620	150	1516
	F	15	420	51	921	148	1353
1959-60	M	5	134	39	435	172	1552
	F	3	120	21	302	158	1424
1960-61	M	-	-	12	222	180	1578
	F	-	-	40	849	165	1335
1961-62	M	6	239	17	385	129	1015
	F	7	345	30	537	151	1099
1962-63	M	11	574	12	157	86	514
	F	13	876	29	482	127	882
1963-64	M	-	-	5	36	56	331
	F	-	-	2	15	132	1062
1964-65	M	-	-	7	130	51	482
	F	-	-	-	-	155	1298
1965-66	M	-	-	6	175	34	216
	F	-	-	14	240	147	103
1966-67	M	-	-	-	-	20	133
	F	-	-	-	-	98	588
1967-68	M	-	-	-	-	45	316
	F	-	-	-	-	80	549

Source: New Brunswick, Department of Health, *Annual Reports* 1954-68. A dash indicates that the treatment was not mentioned in the annual report in question.

was in an industrialized area rather than in the province's political capital. In addition, in two cases, buildings that had previously served other purposes — the treatment of cholera and tuberculosis — were used. Thus, as soon as one scourge was eliminated, it was replaced by another and dealt with in the same manner.

2.2 TREATMENT IN THE COMMUNITY

2.2.1 The Era of Clinics and Special Care Homes

In 1968 a bill aimed at reforming and deinstitutionalizing psychiatric care was tabled in the New Brunswick Legislative Assembly. Emphasis was to be placed on diagnosing patients, treating them and returning them to the community, which would have to have sufficient services at its disposal to house and treat the mentally ill. Later a complete network of psychosocial clinics was set up in every regional centre.

The new legislation, which replaced the Provincial Hospitals Act, went into effect in February 1970. Psychiatric patients, who previously had had no legal recourse, were for the first time given the right to appeal decisions that concerned them. The new law provided for psychiatric services in general hospitals, and some hospitals later set up networks of specialized psychiatric services. Five hospitals now have such services: Saint John Hospital, l'Hôtel-Dieu Hospital in Campbellton, Moncton Hospital, Dr. Everett Chalmers Hospital in Fredericton, and Dr. Georges-L. Dumont hospital in Moncton.

The Department of Health had long been interested in the role that could be played by special care homes in psychiatric treatment. As far back as 1895, the superintendent of the Provincial Hospital of Saint John had gone to Belgium to study the Gheel, a network of homes authorized to take in former inmates of psychiatric institutions. This initiative was highly praised at the time. However, it was only in the late 1960s that the concept surfaced in New Brunswick. Individuals who were considered ready to leave the confines of the institution were placed in special homes. The 1974-75 annual report of the Department of Health commented: "Foster homes and nursing homes might be called our third mental hospital. At the end of 1974, there were 775 patients in these facilities who were previously resident in the psychiatric hospitals."

Thus, one of the reasons the number of patients in the two psychiatric institutions declined after the 1960s was that a new system of care was taking over. The operating costs of the traditional institutions had in-

Figure 4
Mental Health Services in New Brunswick, 1985

Psychiatric hospitals

Restigouche Hospital Center, Campbellton
Centracare, Saint John

General Hospitals

Saint John General Hospital	30 beds
L'Hôtel-Dieu Hospital, Campbellton	14 beds
Moncton Hospital	20 beds
Dr. Everett Chalmers Hospital, Fredericton	30 beds
Dr. Georges-L. Dumont Hospital, Moncton	20 beds

Regional clinics

Region I   - Mental Health Clinic, Moncton
            - Local clinic: Sainte-Anne de Kent
            - Travelling clinic: Shédiac, Sackville & Albert County
Region II   - Mental Health Clinic, Saint John
            - Local clinics: St. Stephen, Sussex
            - Travelling clinics: St. Andrews, Grand Manan
Region III - Mental Health Clinic, Fredericton
            - Local clinic: Woodstock
            - Travelling clinics: Doaktown, McAdam, Fredericton
              Junction, Minto, Oromocto
Region IV   - Mental Health Clinic, Edmundston
            - Local clinic: Grand-Sault
Region V   - Mental Health Clinic, Campbellton
            - Travelling clinics: St. Quentin, Dalhousie
Region VI   - Mental Health Clinic, Bathurst
            - Local clinic: Caraquet
Region VII - Mental Health Clinic, Chatham

Local clinics have a full-time staff and a travelling psychiatrist.
Travelling clinics have no full-time staff, but are visited regularly by
psychiatric workers.

creased considerably, their rate of long-term cure was low (66 per cent of patients were readmitted), and people were losing confidence in institutional treatment.

2.2.2 The Current Situation

As a result of this new direction in institutional psychiatry, the Department of Health decided to open clinics in a number of the province's urban centres. In eight years the number of outpatient clinics quadrupled. However, no special effort was made to ensure that psychiatric care was included in general hospitals, partly because the general hospitals refused to offer services for the mentally ill. As one psychiatrist said, "General hospitals care for the physically ill; the administrators and staff don't want patients who are mentally ill."

New Brunswick currently has two psychiatric hospitals, twelve mental health clinics, six satellite clinics and six mobile clinics. Six general hospitals offer psychiatric services.

NOTES

1. Dorothy Chen, *Historical Facts on the Provincial Hospital* (mimeo., June 1967), p. 15.
2. Michel Foucault, *Madness and Civilization: A History of Insanity in the Age of Reason* (London: Tavistock Publications, 1967), p. 8.
3. Travis Cushing, "Some History of Mental Health in New Brunswick," in: *Report on the Provincial Conference on Mental Health Held by the New Brunswick Division of the Canadian Mental Health Association, Memramcook Institute,* November 12-14, 1976 (Mental Health/New Brunswick and Canadian Mental Health Association, n.d.), p. 1.
4. Foucault, *Madness and Civilization* , p. 45.
5. Georges Devereux, *Essais d'ethnopsychiatrie générale* (Paris: Gallimard, 1970), p. 1.
6. Cushing, "Some History of Mental Health," p. 3.
7. Roger Gentis, *Les murs de l'asile* (Paris: Maspero, 1970), p. 12.
8. Chen, *Historical Facts*, p. 3.
9. John O'Neill, "Le Langage et la décolonisation", *Sociologies et Sociétés* 6, no. 2: 54.
10. Chen, *Historical Facts* , p. 6.
11. Cushing, "Some History of Mental Health," p. 2.
12. R.D. Laing, *The Politics of Experience* (New York: Pantheon Books, 1967), p. 75.

3
The Role of Psychiatry

There is no joy when considering the confinement of a mad person; necessity is the rule. The calamity is in the madness, not in the measure taken. Cure it, if possible; prevent dangerous lapses; that is the duty imposed by the laws of humanity and the preservation of society.
— Casimir Pinel, 1861

Here, we give out electric shocks like aspirin. No one knows exactly what it does to a person ... After six months, we give them more ...
— Resource person on a guided tour, Centracare, 1982

3.1 SOCIAL DEVIANCE AND PSYCHIATRY

Since psychiatry became a medical science, took over the field of mental health, and gained the power to diagnose and treat deviants and deviance, it has been criticized on numerous occasions.

Has "the doctor of the soul" — to go back to the root of the term psychiatrist — measured up to his title? Or has he enmeshed us in a medico-legal labyrinth? Haven't his diagnoses, interpretations and treatments been limited to the individual, and hasn't the social context been ignored? Haven't the people he has identified as being in need of treatment been those who see problems and think in a way that falls outside the norm — outside of what is considered "normal"? Roger Gentis answers this question by saying that we must attack the norm: the norm must be "cured" so that we may eventually *cure life*, as the title of one of his books proclaims.

In his analysis of suicide, Durkheim described the circumstances and social context that lead some people to take their own lives. It may not be out of place to suggest that social problems which are considered purely individual abnormalities, such as certain mental illnesses, are in fact manifestations of these same contextual factors. Thus, the relationship between anomie and suicide should be applicable to mental illness. Although seen by traditional psychiatry as individual deviance, mental illness could actually be the sign of an underlying current or social malaise affecting an individual or a group.

In New Brunswick, for example, three times as many Acadians as Anglophones are diagnosed as suffering from neurosis. How can this fact be explained, if not as a symptom of a social malaise? The anxiety Acadians suffer can be seen as the result of a history of reprisals, domination and repression.

When traditional psychiatry makes a diagnosis, it looks only at the individual, and occasionally at the individual's immediate family and work environment. Diagnosis and treatment follow medical methodology: the "doctor of the soul" deals only with symptoms and individual problems, without going back to their possible roots in the social context.

Roger Bastide has observed that "an increase in the incidence of insanity correlates with a transition from an organic period to a period of crisis." In this sense neurosis, like suicide, is the sign and the expression of a social malaise experienced by an individual or group. Most psychiatrists, however, refuse to consider this possibility. Instead, they overspecialize, limiting themselves to individual diagnosis and treatment even though the cases they see are often no more than the expression of a malaise — the indication of deviance and not the deviance itself.

Michel Foucault provided the historical antecedents of this interpretation of madness, while Roger Bastide noted that Talcott Parsons presented psychiatric deviance as a sociological phenomenon:

Parsons defines deviance as a reluctance or an inability of the ego to internalize certain rules or even to make its behaviour conform to social norms. He lists four possible personality types: the over-conformist, the rebel, the ritualist and the escapist. Although neurotics may be more likely than others to be ritualists or escapists, the point is that deviance is a sociological and not a psychiatric phenomenon.[1]

In this sense, Bastide argues that the normal and the pathological are culturally relative — that there are a number of definitions of "pathological," varying from one culture to another. Continuing the analogy with the analysis of suicide, we could conclude from this that psychiatric deviance can be interpreted as a sign of social anomie.

3.2 PSYCHIATRY AND RELIGION

In the Middle Ages madness was considered a sin, and mad people were not allowed to enter churches. Since the time of Casimir Pinel, however, madness has passed from the domain of sin into the domain of pathology: until recently, mad people were refused admission to general hospitals. When religion was at the foundation of social values, it had the power to exclude. Now that medicine has replaced traditional religion, achieving the dual status of a science and a new religion, it is medicine that has the power to exclude. Medicine excludes and provides care — it excludes to provide care.

Thomas Szasz draws a parallel between the development of medicine and the loss of power by religion. To sum up his thesis, doctors — and psychiatrists in particular — have taken over the power once held by religion, along with the myths that religion upheld. Figure 5 is a summary of Szasz's theory of the relationship between medicine and religion. Szasz concludes from this comparison that "God did not die; He merely disappeared behind the stage of history to don other robes and reemerged as scientist and doctor."[2]

In Quebec, as Françoise Boudreau has eloquently shown, the control that religious orders exercised over asylums was a very important source of political power. What was at stake was not so much the treatment of the mentally ill as the interpretation of mental illness according to religious values: "Curing mad people was a frill...What was important was to save their souls. As the owners of the system, the religious orders had full power to run it without being accountable to anyone."[3]

Madness has continued to be regarded as sacred servitude; only the form has changed. As Michel Foucault wrote:

Freed from his chains but declared criminally and civilly irrespon-sible, excluded from society, the madman is completely enslaved to his doctor, to his doctor's healthy, normal ego, to the ideal of rationality his doctor represents ... Thus while the victim of mental illness is entirely alienated in the real person of his doctor, the doctor dissipates the reality of mental illness in the critical concept of madness.[4]

There has always been a profession to take charge of madness — to explain and exclude it. Formerly, power was represented by the priest and the religious order. Now it comes in the form of the doctor-psychiatrist, the modern-day priest whose role is to interpret and heal our medical and social problems. But only the agents have changed; the approach remains the same.

Thus, it is not the relationship between religion and madness, or between medicine and madness, that must be looked at here. What is fundamental is how power is manifested in various ways in different political and historical contexts. Consequently, Szasz suggests that "people should respect their physicians for their skill but should distrust them for their power."[5]

On this question, Christian Delacampagne reminds us that etym-ologically, *maladie*, the French word for illness, has a cosmic and not an individual meaning:

Its sense is astronomical — a perturbation in the movement of the heavens or the rhythm of the seasons — and hence supra-individual. That is why it was possible to apply it to social phenomena. And it was only as a metaphor that it was shifted from this supra-individual level to the

Figure 5
Characteristics of Religion Compared with Characteristics of Medicine

	Basis	Location	Mediator	Deviance	Sentence	Traditional costume	Territory	Powers
Religion	God	Soul	Priest—instrument of passage from life to death	Sin	Hell	Cassock	Church—no access for mad people	Religious and medical
Medicine	Science	Body	Doctor—instrument of passage from sickness to health and from life to death	Sickness	Death	White coat	General hospital—no access for mad people	Medical and religious

strictly individual level of general medicine. Thus, when psychiatry was constituted as a branch of medicine, the word 'maladie' was extended from general medicine to psychiatry, which structured madness as mental illness, that is to say an individual phenomenon.[6]

3.3 THE INTERPRETIVE POWER OF PSYCHIATRY

Ultimately, what is the role of the psychiatrist? Is he or she not an agent of the powers-that-be, hired to ensure that order reigns? In the seventeenth century, doctors were called the "medical police" because their function was to ensure the growing power and wealth of the monarch. Now they are agents of the power of production and guardians of the established order. Their task is to "cure" the oppressed but not oppression, the individual who revolts but not the revolt itself, the delinquent but not delinquency. They are there essentially to rehabilitate "lost sheep" and make them able to work.

"I asked the police to bring me here [to the psychiatric institution] because I'm out of work," said Mr. X, a forty-six-year-old Anglophone from Charlotte County, in 1971.

Mrs. Y, 52, a housewife, wants to die. To stop her from killing herself, she is admitted (for the eighth time) and given a series of five electroshocks because "she is a danger to herself."

Mr. X, 23, is an unmarried Anglophone from an industrial town whose mother died when he was seven. Afterwards, he had to be placed in twenty-five different foster homes because none of his foster parents could cope with his problem of incontinence. At fourteen, he began to live in institutions. He stayed in six of them before he arrived in the psychiatric hospital on the orders of a judge. His file notes that "this man claims that television is a school for crime and that people who make violent movies should be charged and punished." His psychiatrist commented: "As we can see, this is a person who is always ready to blame others and not himself. Diagnosis: antisocial personality."

Mr. V, 26, an Acadian from Gloucester County: "He lives from day to day, on the fringes of society. He has no permanent home and rejects the traditional values of family, religion and work. He calls himself Acadian and is proud of his heritage; as a result, he claims that he is a member of an oppressed minority. In addition, he denounces religion and the socio-economic ethic of capitalism." Diagnosis: unbalanced personality; a social misfit.

What is the role of psychiatrists if not to take charge of deviants and bring them back to normal, no matter what the cause of the "illness"? Psychiatry is nothing less than a profession that serves the established order, using its power to enforce the norm. According to Robert Nadeau, "the origins of the asylum, the clinic and the prison all involve a change in the way in which power entraps the body itself ... Power produces a system in which knowledge is its instrument."[7]

The basis of traditional psychiatry has been questioned by the anti-psychiatry movement. Through the work of R.D. Laing, David Cooper, Franco Basaglia and Thomas Szasz, in particular, the principles underlying psychiatric institutions — whose development corresponds with that of traditional psychiatry itself—have been shaken, and this has caused the traditional definition of madness to be called into question. We are now witnessing the emergence of a new direction in psychiatry: community psychiatry. It involves a new means of dealing with deviance and a new and more subtle redefinition of target groups. On this subject, Françoise and Robert Castel and Anne Lovell wrote:

Despite a steady stream of innovations on the system's fringes, there is, within the constantly changing borders, a carefully laid-out market in which clients are shifted from one stall to the next. These shifts are determined by the social problems supposedly posed by each client group. Changes in institutional structures, methodologies and theoretical models are governed by the growing demand for services. All the current efforts to redefine problems, redistribute skills, and cope with "crises of adjustment" in the American mental health care system come to the fore, as we shall see, with the advent of new client groups that had previously lain beyond the system's reach.[8]

As a result of the pressures exerted on it, psychiatry is abandoning the traditional institutional model and moving towards community psychiatry. Thus New Brunswick's Department of Health could say, as noted earlier, that nursing homes are "our third mental hospital." Can this statement have any other meaning than that deinstitutionalization is a sign of adaptation, not of change? It is the status quo in disguise.

NOTES

1. Roger Bastide, *The Sociology of Mental Disorder* (London: Routledge and Kegan Paul, 1972), p. 57.
2. Thomas Szasz, *The Theology of Medicine* (Baton Rouge: Louisiana State University Press, 1977), p. 3.
3. Françoise Boudreau, *De l'asile à la santé mentale* (Montreal: Editions Saint-Martin, 1984), pp. 52 - 54.
4. Michel Foucault, *Histoire de la folie à l'âge classique* (Paris: Gallimard, 1972), p. 529, and *Madness and Civilization* (London: Tavistock Publications Ltd., 1965), p. 277.
5. Szasz, *Theology of Medicine* , p. xxii.
6. Christian Delacampagne, *Antipsychiatrie, les voies du sacré* (Paris: Grasset, 1974), p. 169.
7. Robert Nadeau, "Michel Foucault ou le développement impitoyable," *Critère* no. 13 (March 1976), pp. 190, 195.
8. Robert Castel, Françoise Castel, and Anne Lovell, *The Psychiatric Society* (New York: Columbia University Press, 1982), p. xx.

4

Working Hypotheses: Involuntary Hospitalization, Ethnic Origin and Industrialization

"Society rids itself of all those who have slipped outside the world of 'production' and 'consumption.'"

— Roger Gentis

4.1 INDUSTRIALIZATION AND EXCLUSION

According to the political economist Jacques Attali, psychiatry in the industrial era can be interpreted as corresponding to the third stage of evil in human history. In the first stage, evil was a mark of God, and religion was the therapist, while in the second, evil was a mark of the body, with police forces playing the major role. In the industrial era, evil has been the mark of machines.

In this stage, the body is a machine and therefore must produce. Otherwise it must be treated — this is the role of medicine — or excluded indefinitely because it is harmful to the cycle of production-consumption-reproduction. This exclusion affects not only the mentally ill, but also a variety of other social groups and people diagnosed as deviants. The mad are excluded along with the delinquent, the elderly, the sick, political deviants, drug addicts, alcoholics ... According to the French writer René Lenoir, "one fifth of the population of France is now considered socially maladapted and excluded and this percentage is constantly increasing."[1]

Statistics Canada says that "one of every eight Canadians can expect to be hospitalized for a mental illness at least once during his or her lifetime ... Between 10 per cent and 30 per cent of the population have some form of mental illness, depending on the perceptions and definitions of the various disorders in this group."[2]

In the industrial society in which we live, there must be production, consumption and exchange. What about those members of society who are unable or unwilling to accept and internalize these values and to produce in the commercial sense of the term? Because they fulfill no social role in terms of production, have no useful labour power, and do not make an acceptable contribution ideologically and economically, all sorts of reasons are found to reject them; they have no say in the matter, and are either shut away or simply ignored. David Riesman has used the concept of anomie to sum up the possibilities open to modern humanity as it confronts the values of industrial society: "Modern industrial society has driven great numbers of people into anomie, and produced a wan conformity in others."[3]

It is necessary to get rid of deviants and mad people; but more than that, madness itself must be eliminated. Mad people are institutionalized, but above all, madness is the target. This explains the development of an entire structure and network of services and laws, all leading towards the psychiatric institution.

Who are the mad? Since the time of Descartes, the mad have been those who have lost their reason. Reason plays the predominant role and even characterizes the industrial, technological and commercial era in which we now live, the era of capitalism.

Individuals become commodities exchanged on the basis of their commercial value and their capacity for labour. Those who do not accept these values and cannot produce through labour are generally excluded. This norm is essential to the development of capitalist society, and psychiatry, claiming a basis in science— itself based on reason and representing a guarantee of progress — ensures that it is respected. The work of Erving Goffman in particular has amply demonstrated the contribution made by totalitarian institutions in disseminating and monitoring adherence to the dominant ideology.[4]

In this sense, psychiatric institutions and their agents play an active role in the production process by ensuring the continued hegemony of the dominant ideology.

4.2 INTEGRATION OR CONFINEMENT

Exclusion by reason of insanity is part of the particular historical context of the development of an industrial and commercial society that promotes particular values and ideas about the socioeconomic role of human beings — in other words, a social model. In this type of society, industrial centres emerge. The hinterland adapts to this development, going along with the demands of the industrial centres which coordinate and control economic activity, development and planning. This process creates adjustment problems for dominated groups, which cannot remain isolated indefinitely from the pull of the industrial centre. Sooner or later, they have to submit and accommodate to it, as the centre, in the name of progress, strengthens its hold on the hinterland.

As early as 1851, according to Dr. John Waddell, director of the asylum at Saint John, industrialization and economic progress were contributing to a growth in the number of people who were mentally ill. Speaking of the consequences of railway construction, he made the following comment:

The new impulse which such great works will impart to the latent energies of a hitherto quiet population, will contribute largely, I have no doubt, to the production of mental disease. It is probable that to this cause, more than to any other, may be attributed the great increase of insanity in those countries where Railroads and other great public works are revolutionizing the business transactions, and overstimulating the energies of the people.[5]

For a long time the Acadians, by choice or by circumstance, remained outside this kind of development and kept their marginal, traditional lifestyle. They lived by fishing, hunting and farming in a rural environment that contained little that would attract the architects of development. However, because of the maritime and mineral resources of northeastern New Brunswick, Acadia found itself suddenly catapulted into the industrial and technological twentieth century.

It should be noted that Premier Louis Robichaud's plan, in the 1960s, contributed to the integration of the Acadian population of the northeastern and southeastern parts of the province. The main element of this plan was the equal opportunity program which promoted the penetration of regions which until then had been marginal and industrially and technologically underdeveloped by economic liberalism.

This perspective provides the basis for a first working hypothesis, involving the relationship between exclusion on the one hand and lack of integration into industrialization on the other.

4.3 FIRST WORKING HYPOTHESIS: INDUSTRIALIZATION AND EXCLUSION

The industrial era favours norms and behaviour corresponding to its own particular social values. This can be seen clearly by looking at the kinds of individuals admitted to psychiatric institutions and the reasons for admitting them. Table 8 shows that:

• the five provinces with a higher rate of involuntary admission than the national average are, in descending order, British Columbia, Alberta, New Brunswick, Nova Scotia and Prince Edward Island;

• the provinces outside of Central Canada have the highest proportion of involuntary admissions;

Table 8
Percentage of Admissions That Are Involuntary by
Province and Sex, 1981-82

Province	Men (%)	Women (%)
Newfoundland	(not available)	
Prince Edward Island	52	30
Nova Scotia	51	40
New Brunswick	(57% men and women)	
Quebec	30	20
Ontario	38	33
Manitoba	(not available)	
Saskatchewan	22	14
Alberta	64	68
British Columbia	89	88
Canada	42	34

Source: Statistics Canada

• the provinces outside of Central Canada have the highest proportion of involuntary admissions;

• in every province except Alberta, the percentage of involuntary admissions is higher for men than for women.

4.4 INVOLUNTARY TREATMENT

Involuntary hospitalization is only the first stage in the treatment of the individual admitted to a psychiatric institution. Other stages of treatment are also forced on patients who, in many cases, do not agree to these treatments any more than they agree to be admitted to the hospital in the first place.

Furthermore, the consent form used upon admission authorizes medical personnel to "carry out the necessary examinations and to prescribe medication." Figure 6 shows the form still in use today. How can treatment be effective when the person involved is not consulted either in the choice of treatment or in how it is administered?

While the subject of involuntary treatment is much broader than the question of involuntary admission alone, only admission will be dealt with here. At the same time, it is worth noting that involuntary treatment is an embarrassing problem for the psychiatric profession, and not necessarily

AUTHORIZATION FOR EXAMINATION, ADMINISTRATION OF MEDICATIONS AND RELEASE OF INFORMATION

DECLARATION IN CASE OF MEDICALLY UNAUTHORIZED DISCHARGE

AUTHORIZATION TO BE COMPLETED UPON SUBMISSION

(THIS SECTION MUST BE COMPLETED FOR EACH PATIENT UPON ADMISSION. IS PATIENT IS ADMITTED AGAINST HIS WILL AND NO AUTHORIZED PERSON IS AVAILABLE, FORM 1 MUST BE COMPLETED.)

II, THE UNDERSIGNED, HEREBY AUTHORIZE ALL HOSPITAL PHYSICIANS INVOLVED IN MY TREATMENT TO CARRY OUT THE NECESSARY EXAMINATIONS AND TO PRESCRIBE MEDICATION, IF REQUIRED. I ALSO AUTHORIZE THE RELEASE OF RELEVANT INFORMATION TO OTHER STAFF MEMBERS AS REQUIRED BY TREATMENT.

_____   _____
DATE   *SIGNATURE

*AUTHORIZATION MUST BE SIGNED BY THE PATIENT, OR, IN THE CASE OF A MINOR, BY THE PARENT OR LEGAL GUARDIAN HAVING THE APPROPRIATE LEGAL AUTHORITY. IN THE CASE OF A PERSON WHO IS PHYSICALLY OR MENTALLY DISABLED TO SUCH A DEGREE AS TO BE INCAPABLE OF GIVING CONSENT, AUTHORIZATION MUST COME FROM NEXT OF KIN.

advantageous for the patient "cared for" in this way.

It is clear that if those directly concerned were given the choice of being treated in a psychiatric institution or not, the asylums would empty in a minute. Abolishing the practice of involuntary admission and treatment without consent would seriously compromise the psychiatric profession. Table 9 illustrates this situation by summarizing data for New Brunswick's psychiatric institutions.

A mad person who becomes the centre of attention and a distraction implicitly contradicts the values of industrial society and the idea of socially acceptable work. This is why such a person must be excluded in one way or another. An industrialized world will not easily tolerate deviants who are a disturbance and call the system of production into question by their very presence. This model for dealing with madness has also been applied to a number of other marginal groups. The elderly, the unemployed and the handicapped have suffered the same fate as the mentally ill — management by exclusion.

Unproductive units within the nuclear family must provide for their own needs, not an easy task under present socioeconomic conditions. Otherwise, they must depend on institutions of care to help them survive. This explains the marginalization and exclusion of the groups mentioned above. As Henri-Jacques Stiker has written:

To live in families as they are currently conceived, habitats as they are currently constructed, and corporations as they currently organize time and space, people must cut themselves off from old people and sometimes from young ones, entrust their children in trouble to specialists, and exclude the weak and infirm from their homes. Any weakness, any deviance, any failure of adaptation is incompatible with the organization of daily life and especially of urban life.[6]

The "mentally ill" thus become one of the casualties of the growth of our society and the direction it is taking. Because they are not productive and are unable to adapt to the system, they become its victims. Starting out as deviants, they become "mad" once they cross the threshold of the psychiatric institution. By targeting them, it becomes possible to "express as an individual phenomenon a reality that has its origin in the pattern of the collectivity," as Jean Duvignaud has described it.[7] In this sense, any form of disequilibrium will generate a social disturbance, the indications and consequences of which can be found in the individual.

Table 9
Percentage of Admissions That Are Involuntary
New Brunswick, 1974-84

Hospital	Year										
	1974	1975	1976	1977	1978	1979	1980	1981	1982	1983	1984
Restigouche Hospital Center	52	56	55	54	55	56	57	53	58	54	56
Centracare	70	63	53	62	63	73	63	56	61	54	59

Sources: New Brunswick Department of Health, *Annual Reports*; Archives of the institutions

4.5 SECOND WORKING HYPOTHESIS: ETHNIC ORIGIN AND INVOLUNTARY HOSPITALIZATION

For as long as they have coexisted, the various groups living in New Brunswick have fought either to maintain the status quo or to improve their individual or collective lot. This process can be seen in the areas of health, education, the justice system and everyday life in general.

For a long time, studies and reports have shown that inequalities among ethnic groups in New Brunswick continue to exist, and in some cases are even growing. This is the case in spite of the social programs that have been implemented in an attempt to reduce these disparities. We have already seen that, historically, the different ethnic groups developed unevenly and enjoyed an unequal share of power. Changes in the names of some of the province's industrial towns can be interpreted in this light. The town of Petit-Sault became Edmundston in 1850 when the governor of the province, Sir Edmund Head, visited there (the name Edmundston comes from "Edmund's Town"). Saint-Pierre became Bathurst in 1826, in honour of Lord Bathurst, the colonial secretary. Pointe Sainte-Anne became Fredericton in 1785 when the Loyalists came to live there. Before 1766, the city of Moncton was called "Le Coude"; its present name comes from Lieutenant-Colonel Robert Monkton who, at the time of the Deportation in 1755, seized Fort Beauséjour, the last French bastion in Acadia.

On the other hand, Saint John, a Loyalist stronghold since 1783, kept its historic name, which owed its origin to the fact that Champlain sailed up the St. John River (which flows through the city of the same name) on June 24, 1604, the feast day of St. John the Baptist. Elsewhere, regions inhabited by Acadians often kept native names (such as Shédiac, Mada-waska, Tracadie, and Miscou) or took their names from the Catholic church (Saint-André, Saint-Arthur, Sainte-Anne, and the like). The names of towns are a sign of who controls them, a sign of who belongs there, and a reflection of their identity.

Once control was established, political stability was maintained by promoting change through cooperation. This was the bon-ententisme so favoured by the Acadian elite (see chapter 1). Traditionally, Anglophone leaders worked towards improving the lot of their own kind, while Acadian leaders placed themselves at the service of both language communities. A biography of the prominent Acadian jurist Sir Pierre Armand Landry points out that he was "au service de deux peuples" (at the service of two peoples); indeed, this was the title of the biography.[8] Today, in the 1980s, the unequal structure is manifested in several ways:

• While 36.1 per cent of the New Brunswick population is of French ethnic origin, only 15 per cent of senior civil service positions are held by Francophones.

• Only 6 per cent of trials in the Supreme Court, Court of Appeal and County Court were held in French in 1978-79, even though the judicial system was officially bilingual.

• A report published in 1981 described the language situation in the Department of Health:

The linguistic image of the upper levels of the Department of Health is almost exclusively Anglophone. The deputy ministers and the heads of the four divisions are all Anglophone. In addition, none of the leading positions within the most important divisions are occupied by Francophone civil servants. In fact, the only services run by Francophones are financial services for special care homes and construction services for sanitary establishments, both in the Administration Division. This situation is all the more serious, in our opinion, in that it is precisely at these upper levels that the direction and implementation of health policies are decided.[9]

• The same study shows that in the area of specialized care, Francophone hospitals in New Brunswick receive 12.8 per cent of the budget while Anglophone hospitals receive 87.2 per cent.

• Looking at the number of doctors as a proportion of the population for the two language groups in New Brunswick leads to similar conclusions: the English-language population is served by two and half times as many doctors as the French-speaking population.

In respect to psychiatric institutions and mental health, institutional unilingualism has provoked a long and heated — and, for the Acadian population, frustrating — debate. Until 1954, the only psychiatric institution was the one in Saint John, which is now called Centracare. English was the language used there on every level. A number of complaints were brought against the institution, one of which concerned a Francophone patient who was apparently beaten to death by an Anglophone employee. In an effort to verify the rumours about the kind of care provided by the institution, a journalist from Montreal, Kenneth Johnstone, worked as a guard in the institution. He subsequently published first-hand accounts accusing the psychiatric hospital of mistreating its patients. These scandalous allegations forced the government to set up the Baxter Royal Commission in 1945. The commission recommended, among other things, that a psychiatric institution for Francophones be set up in the northern part of the province. This hospital opened in 1954, but from the beginning it has functioned almost exclusively in English, with predominantly Anglophone administrators and staff.

The struggle that was later waged to obtain services in French was long and arduous; indeed, it is not yet over. When he was forced to leave the province in 1976 for reasons he could not state, Dr. Ashley Robin, who practised psychiatry in Campbellton, expressed the opinion that "if the vast majority of patients can express themselves in both languages, it would not be out of line for psychiatric personnel to try to improve their French."[10] A study of the doctors and psychiatrists who have worked in this hospital in the first 27 years of its existence (1954-1981) shows that only 24 per cent of the psychiatrists and 21 per cent of the doctors could speak French.[11] A look at the country of origin of the psychiatrists makes it clear that professionals from foreign countries have been brought in to treat members of Canadian minority cultures. Barely 20 per cent of the psychiatrists are of Canadian origin and only four psychiatrists have Acadian surnames — this in an institution that claims to serve New Brunswick's Acadian population.

What have been the consequences of this situation? A 1968 report by M.T.D. Associates formally noted the case of a Francophone who chose to take her own life rather than return to an institution where she was rebuked by her psychiatrist because she was unable to understand him when he spoke in English. In 1973, the hospital staff was accused of criminal negligence following the death of a patient. The English-language Campbellton Tribune described the situation in the following terms:

Two deaths and a batch of resignations, including that of the acting clinical director, are the latest espisodes in the distasteful history of the hospital in recent years. The hospital, with 600 mentally ill patients, is now operating with a medical staff consisting of a single general practitioner, along with an occasional visit of a trained psychiatrist from Fredericton [300 kilometres away]. Many of their staff members also are simply recruited off the street and given only whatever training is possible on the job.[12]

A staff member at the Restigouche Hospital Center reported that in 1983, a Francophone "patient" had to remain hospitalized an extra year because when his case came up for annual review, the language barrier prevented the psychiatrist from understanding that his family was prepared to take him home.

The power structure is reflected in institutions that serve the public. In fact, the struggle for equality in mental health services is only one illustration of political, economic and social conflict among ethnic groups living in the same province. This leads to a number of questions regarding involuntary hospitalization. What is the situation for the various ethnic groups? Do they have the same conception of normality and abnormality, or does each have its own values? Is it therefore possible to say that there is no universally held definition of madness in New Brunswick? Even if the laws, services, and medical and institutional structures are identical, is it not possible that people are admitted to psychiatric institutions for ethnic rather than medical or legal reasons — especially if their admission is involuntary? Is it not possible that each group rejects from its culture everything that does not conform to the norms by which it lives? Is it not also possible that leaders control deviance by enforcing a universal standard of behaviour in a province whose different groups have major distinguishing features?

If the answer to these questions is yes, it means that each of the three groups has its own definition of what is acceptable, its own criteria for what is marginal and what is not, and its own relationship to "madness." In other words, each group uses the psychiatric institution for its own particular purposes, but the institution and its staff work on the basis of psychiatric principles that are considered universal.

A good example is an Acadian woman who told her psychiatrist she had "butterflies in her stomach." The psychiatrist, who came from outside Canada, made an immediate diagnosis: she was psychotic. Yet, at certain times, all Acadians will have "butterflies in their stomachs"!

In our exploration of how the unacceptable, and rejection because of madness, may be defined in ethnic terms, the following hypothesis will be used as a guide: *Unacceptable behaviour leading to exclusion in a psychiatric institution includes characteristics peculiar to the three ethnic groups that are the subject of this study: the Irish, the Loyalists and the Acadians.* According to this hypothesis, some people are excluded and put away in psychiatric institutions because of a particular cultural conception of what is unacceptable. If this is true, it would be possible for a person living in a certain milieu to be considered mentally ill, while the same person living elsewhere in the same province, with the same laws, the same policies and the same institutions, would be considered normal. This raises the possibility that Acadians forced to integrate into an industrial society would be obliged to conform to "English" criteria of normality that are different from the norms prevailing in their own sociohistoric context.

Referring to Africa, Roy Preiswerk notes that "for decades, the elites have been fascinated by the program of assimilation that consists of offering Africans social equality on the condition that they be prepared to give up their own cultural identity."[13] This was a promise the dominant group often made to the Acadian elite, and even more to the Acadian population. The stage we are now in is one of self-colonization, to use Preiswerk's term. The Acadian elite has confidence in this strategy and has internalized it. It believes in a better future based on economic-political liberalism giving equal opportunities to all the groups in the province. It has taken upon itself the responsibility of dangling this myth of equality before the Acadian population, thus maintaining a structure of domination through an elite power game.

Designated by society as being subject to confinement, the patient who is admitted involuntarily becomes an object of research. The initial diagnosis is social rather than medical, and in this sense, the diagnosis is culturally determined. The powerful in psychiatry and the powerful in society pass "patients" back and forth to each other, and these patients fulfill different purposes for each power group.

NOTES

1. René Lenoir, *Les exclus* (Paris: Seuil, 1974), p. 9.
2. Canada, Statistics Canada, *One of Eight: Mental Illness in Canada* (Ottawa: Supply and Services, 1981).
3. David Riesman, *The Lonely Crowd* (New Haven: Yale University Press, 1961), p. 257.
4. See especially Erving Goffman, *Asylums* (Garden City, N.Y.: Anchor Books, 1961).
5. New Brunswick, Legislative Assembly, *Report of the Medical Superintendent for 1851*, Appendix.
6. Henri-Jacques Stiker, *Corps infirmes et sociétés* (Paris: Aubier, 1982), p. 207.
7. Jean Duvignaud, *L'Anomie: hérésie et subversion* (Paris: Anthropos, 1973), pp. 21-22.
8. Della M. M. Stanley, *Au service de deux peuples* (Moncton: Editions d'Acadie, 1977).
9. André Braen, *La Santé au Nouveau-Brunswick* (Moncton: Société des Acadiens du Nouveau-Brunswick, 1981), p. 107.
10. Dr. Ashley Robin, unpublished letter to the New Brunswick Department of Health.
11. R. Sirois and S. Fortier, *Problèmes linguistiques de l'hôpital psychiatrique de Campbellton*, unpublished study presented to the Department of Social Work, Université de Moncton, December 1981.
12. Campbellton *Tribune*, July 4, 1973.
13. Roy Preiswerk, *Le savoir et le faire* (Paris: Presses Universitaires de France, 1975), p. 64.

5
The Unequal Burden of Involuntary Hospitalization

The mental hospital is just such a place where the means and ends of human action seem out of joint, and where myths and collective beliefs exist in order to maintain a collective fiction: that treatment and discharge are the central goals of the hospital. This fiction is necessary to allow the society to deal with the fact that it rejects some of its members; it is necessary for hospital staff in order to maintain their favourable self-concepts; and it is even necessary for the patients in order to avoid accepting the harsh reality of a lifetime in the hospital.

—Robert Perrucci

Note: This chapter was previously published in the *Revue de l'Université de Moncton* in 1984. I would like to thank the editors for permission to reprint it.

The term "involuntary hospitalization" refers to the forcible admission to a psychiatric institution of any person whose behaviour is considered unacceptable by a given community, and more specifically by the justice and/or medical system. A number of writers have described it as an attack on the personal freedom of individuals who often are not ill but simply do not act or think according to the social norms accepted by the majority. In New Brunswick, the Mental Health Act of 1976 provides for four ways of admitting an individual to a psychiatric institution involuntarily:

• Any policeman or other officer of the law who observes that an individual is "apparently suffering from mental disorder and acting in a manner that in a normal person would be disorderly" can take that individual to "to an appropriate place where he may be detained for medical examination." (article 10 a and b)

• Any citizen "who believes that another person is suffering from mental disorder, and should be examined in the interests of his own safety or the safety of others" can so inform a judge of the provincial court, who can issue an order for the individual to be examined. (article 9 (1))

• Any doctor who declares that an individual "suffers from mental disorder of a nature or degree so as to require hospitalization in the interests of his own safety or the safety of others" and signs a form to this effect can have that individual admitted to a psychiatric institution for a maximum thirty-day examination period. After this initial period, the status of the hospitalized individual must be reviewed unless the institution's authorities consider him a danger to himself or others. The majority of cases (about 80 per cent) of involuntary hospitalization in New Brunswick fall into this third category.

• There are also situations where the mental health of individuals who appear in court is questioned by judicial authorities: "Where the presiding judge has reason to believe that a person who appears before him charged with or convicted of an offence suffers from mental disorder, he may order that person to attend a psychiatric facility for examination." (article 14 (1))

As well, the Criminal Code (chapter C-34) provides that an individual who has been found guilty of a crime can be sent to a psychiatric institution on grounds of his or her mental state.

The law is somewhat vague on the question of reasons for involuntary hospitalization. What does the phrase "suffers from mental disorder of a nature or degree so as to require hospitalization in the interests of his own safety or the safety of others" mean? What criteria does an officer of the law use to decide that a person is behaving in "a manner that in a normal person would be disorderly"? The provision that anyone "who believes that another person is suffering from mental disorder" can recommend that a person be examined may provide society with a necessary form of protection, but it can also be subject to abuse.

In Canada, there have been few studies of involuntary hospitalization and the reasons for it. Marc-Adélard Tremblay and Gérald Louis Gold, in one study, and Charles Hughes and his colleagues in another, have examined the cultural aspects of deviance in certain specific groups. Robert Mayer and Henri Dorvil have studied historical and political questions in the Quebec context. Recent studies by Anne Paquet-Deehy and her colleagues have looked at the differences between mental illness in men and women. As well, in a previous historical study of mental health in New Brunswick, I have raised some questions about rates of involuntary hospitalization and the influence of psychiatric experts (many of them non-Canadian) on users of psychiatric services.[1]

This chapter presents the results of research carried out on this question. The tables and accompanying observations show that interpretation of the law, which should theoretically apply to all New Brunswick citizens in the same way, in fact varies enormously from place to place. The following variables are discussed:

- involuntary hospitalization and ethnic group;
- involuntary hospitalization and marital status;
- involuntary hospitalization and sex;
- involuntary hospitalization and occupation;
- involuntary hospitalization and proximity to an institution.

In looking at involuntary hospitalization by ethnic group, particular attention will be paid to Acadians in New Brunswick to determine whether they interpret mental health legislation in a particular way. To this end, the percentage of involuntary admissions for Acadians will be compared to those for other groups in the province.

5.1 METHOD OF ADMISSION AND ETHNIC ORIGIN

Table 10 compares the percentage of involuntary admissions for a number of ethnic groups living in the province of New Brunswick. In the table, the term "English" includes all English-speaking people except the Irish and the Scots; these two groups could be listed separately because they were identified separately on the psychiatric institution's admission forms. However, the files did not provide any means of identifying Loyalists, and so they have been included in the "English" category in this part of the study.

The following observations can be made from the table. Fifty per cent of the Irish and Scots admitted were hospitalized involuntarily. The "others" category shows about the same percentage, while 61.9 per cent of the people in the "English" category were admitted involuntarily. For Acadians, the percentage was over 70 per cent; Acadian society, which is more traditional, seems to apply stricter norms to its deviants.

A comment is in order here on the overall organization of health care services in New Brunswick, and especially its ethnic dimension. In 1980, the provincial Department of Health had twenty-two administrators, of whom twenty had English surnames.[2] When this study was completed in 1981, only one of the four psychiatrists practising at the psychiatric hospital in Campbellton was considered bilingual; the others were unable to speak French. This situation has changed since 1983, when five Francophone psychiatrists were hired by the board of directors of the Campbellton hospital (now the Restigouche Hospital Center). It was the first time in its thirty years of existence that the hospital had a French-language psychiatric team.

The problems created by an "English-style" administrative structure are considerable. Anglophones were in control of every level of the hospital hierarchy at the Restigouche Hospital Center which, it must be recalled, was built for the Francophone community in the early 1950s. Before that, Francophones were committed to the psychiatric institution in Saint John and had to adapt to treatment in English there.

This is the context for the events related in the file of Mr. X, an Acadian from Kent County, admitted to the Saint John hospital in 1940 at the age of thirty-seven.

1940: Admitted to the Provincial Hospital in Saint John: "The patient is frightened and uncooperative."

1942: "No change. He is confused and unenergetic."

Table 10
Percentage of Admissions That Are Involuntary
by Ethnic Origin, 1956-81

Ethnic group	Number of files	%
Scottish	10	50
Irish	36	51.4
English	211	61.9
Acadian	284	70.9
Others	44	48.5
Total sample	**585**	**64.9**

1952: "This individual seems to have trouble understanding English. However, he is cooperative and seems happy to be here."

1970: "He likes to work with his hands. However, he is not very clean and dresses sloppily. He only speaks French."

1972: "His chances for rehabilitation are almost nonexistent. In psychiatric terms, he's a 'burn-out.'"

1977: "Not yet ready to be released. Hospital treatment must continue."

1982: At the time of the study, Mr. X was still in hospital; he had been there for forty-two years.

In his book *Cinq ans de trop*, Pierre Godin describes what Acadians experienced at the Restigouche Hospital Center. He recounts the following incident:

I never saw a film presented in French. In addition, the person in charge was a unilingual Anglophone. But was he working for himself or for the patients? For 85 per cent of these old people as well as other patients were Francophones, and 50 per cent of them didn't understand a word of English. One day I wrote a report in French only. You should have seen their reaction. These culturally handicapped people didn't understand any of it, and they never forgave me for it.[3]

The Société des Acadiens du Nouveau-Brunswick made the question of language in this hospital its main concern, particularly in the 1970s. After a long and hard battle a number of changes were made in terms of language, organization of patient care, and patient services.

Because of their history and socioeconomic position, Acadians live in a state of alienation. Only the elite participates in the economic and political power structure, and in return has had to abandon its nationalist and cultural aspirations. The oppression of Acadians in the psychiatric domain is added proof of their alienation and makes it even more tragic.

5.2 MODE OF ADMISSION AND MARITAL STATUS

Five classifications of marital status appeared in the records used to collect data for this study: single, married, separated, divorced and widowed. While the overall proportion of involuntary admissions in this study was 64.4 per cent, widows and widowers were admitted involuntarily at a rate of just over 75 per cent, as shown in figure 7. In this study, the rate for married people roughly coincided with the average, while separated and divorced people had the lowest percentage of involuntary admissions.

At first glance, figure 7 seems to show that marriage is a stabilizing factor, in the sense that married people were admitted involuntarily less often than single people, widows and widowers. This is precisely the conclusion arrived at by Rodney Riley and Alex Richman, who have studied these variables in New Brunswick. "Marriage favours the mental health *of the couple* and protects it against the risks of mental illness. There is extensive documentation to substantiate this statement."[5]

However, further analysis shows that marriage is a stabilizing factor primarily for men. Figure 8 adds the sex of those admitted involuntarily as a third variable, and shows that at 66.7 per cent, the percentage of married women admitted involuntarily is above average, while the percentage for married men is below average at 59.9 per cent.

Furthermore, in all other cases — single, separated, divorced and widowed — the percentage of involuntary admissions is lower for women than for men. This reinforces the conclusion that the institution of marriage appears to benefit men, at least in respect to involuntary hospitalization. They are involuntarily hospitalized more often in all cases, except when they are married. Durkheim reached similar conclusions in his study of the relationship among marriage, gender and suicide.

The higher proportion of married women who enter the psychiatric system is probably primarily the result of their relatively marginalized position in the home and in society. The structure of the family in New Brunswick is markedly patriarchal and conservative and can thus lead to people becoming imprisoned in their respective roles.[6] In her satirical play

Figure 7
Percentage of Admissions That Are
Involuntary by Marital Status, 1956-81

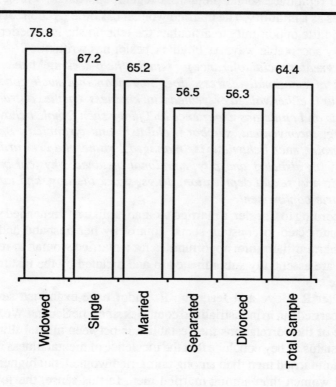

Femme ta boîte*, the Acadian writer-director Monique LeBlanc uses Evangéline as a recurring symbol of martyrdom. This symbol of patience, submissiveness and suffering has no male equivalent.

The married woman who enters the world of madness appears to be subject to increased discrimination. Some doctors — perhaps unconsciously — reproduce social prejudices regarding madness. These doctors will also reproduce social prejudices regarding women, whom society perceives as a minority. The married woman has little freedom of expression and little opportunity to articulate the tension she is experiencing in a socially acceptable way. As Phyllis Chesler has written:

The greater social tolerance for female "help-seeking" behaviour, or displays of emotional distress, does not mean that such conditioned behaviour is either valued or treated with kindness. On the contrary. Both husbands and clinicians experience and judge such female behaviour as annoying, inconvenient, stubborn, childish, and tyrannical. Beyond a certain point, such behaviour is "managed," rather than rewarded: it is treated with disbelief and pity, emotional distance, physical brutality, economic and sexual deprivation, drugs, shock therapy, and long-term psychiatric confinement.[7]

According to Chesler, a married woman, unlike an unmarried woman, can be subjected to constant social control by her husband and others around her. Furthermore, opportunities for a married woman to relax and unwind are essentially subordinated to and dictated by the institution of marriage.[8]

Walter R. Gove and Jeannette F. Tudor have examined seventeen studies carried out in industrialized countries since the Second World War, and one of the correlations they establish is between mental illness and marital status. They conclude that the incidence of mental illness is higher among unmarried men than among unmarried women, but higher among married women than among married men. In this sense, the following statement by Anne Paquet-Deehy and her colleagues is relevant to the Acadian population in general as a disadvantaged group, and specifically to Acadian women:

Women show more of the symptoms of mental illness than men because of the social role that has devolved on them in our modern industrialized societies. We must look for the explanation for women's emotional problems in the differentiated roles that they are required to

---

*A word play on the expression "shut your mouth" (or "shut up"), which becomes "woman, shut your mouth.".

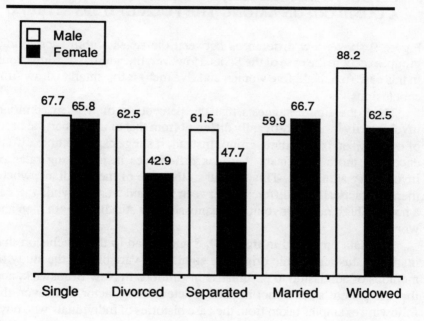

Figure 8
Percentage of Admissions That Are Involuntary
by Sex and Marital Status, 1956-81

*play in relation to men. Most women are called upon to play a single basic
role in their lives, that of housewife, while men can always find two sources
of self-worth — their family and their work. If a woman doesn' t fully reach
her potential by staying at home, where can she go without being made to
feel guilty and regarded as frustrated and selfish?*[10]

If we accept that married women live in a context of structural
oppression, and that Acadian women suffer double oppression, ethnic and
marital, we should examine our data regarding married Acadian women
to see whether they reflect this situation.

5.3 INVOLUNTARY ADMISSION, SEX AND ETHNIC ORIGIN: A COMPARISON AMONG THE FOUR GROUPS STUDIED

Figure 9 shows few differences between the sexes within each ethnic
group, except in the case of the Scots. However, the number of admissions
in this case (ten in all, five women and five men) is too small to draw firm
conclusions.

Thus, the figure suggests that the percentage of women admitted
involuntarily is not significantly different from that of men when the basis
of comparison is the ethnic group. Instead, it suggests that ethnic differences are more significant than sex differences in predicting rates of
involuntary admission. This is clear in the case of the Acadians, where
there is practically no difference between men and women, while there is
a notably high rate of involuntary admission for Acadians, both men and
women.

The data presented in figures 7, 8 and 9 lead to the conclusion that
marital status and ethnic origin are significant variables in the study of
methods of admission to psychiatric institutions in New Brunswick, and
that the patient's sex is not in itself a determining factor. However, the
following examples taken from the case histories of individuals who have
been patients in psychiatric institutions illustrate the situation of hospitalized married women.

Mrs. W, aged twenty-one, married, a housewife, from an Acadian
family of seventeen children: "When she was young, she was beaten and
mistreated by her alcoholic father; he tried to rape her; he threw her down
a staircase. She often dreams she is being murdered and emits loud cries.
She is afraid of the dark." Her diagnosis: personality disorder, hysteria.

Noteworthy here is the way women and their problems are regarded.
The diagnosis of her condition blames her for a situation for which she was

Figure 9
Percentage of Admissions That Are Involuntary
by Sex and Ethnic Origin, 1956-81

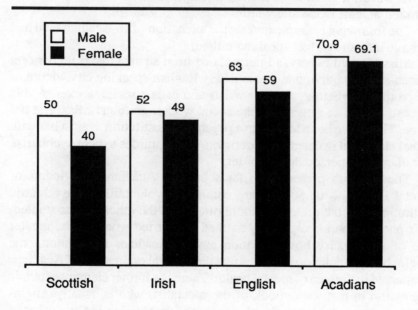

not entirely responsible. She is being hospitalized to bring her back to "normality" through diagnosis followed by treatment.

Mrs. X, aged forty-five, Acadian, a housewife, is admitted involuntarily in 1961 for a second bout of post-partum psychosis. Here is what her psychiatrist notes: "Mrs. X was admitted once before and was given electroshock treatment because she was suffering from post-partum psychosis. I do not think at this point that this slender woman, who is suffering from malnutrition and is excessively thin, is psychotic. She has had a dozen children and lives in deplorable economic conditions, and her husband is unemployed."

However, a close look at the records reveals that this woman was admitted at least twice afterwards.

The following example reveals the alienation of an Acadian who had to move into an English-speaking milieu:

Miss V, aged twenty, a Francophone from an area that is 95 per cent French-speaking, living in a completely English-speaking city, victim of a rape the year before, slits her wrists and calls a social worker. At his request, the police rather than the social worker go to get Miss V at her home. They have her admitted to a psychiatric institution against her will. "I feel alone and isolated in Fredericton," she confides to her psychiatrist. Her diagnosis: personality disorder.

The statistics presented so far show that Acadians are victims of mental illness — or at least are confined involuntarily in psychiatric institutions on that pretext — more often than the other groups studied. This phenomenon is especially marked in married women. The greater rate of involuntary hospitalization among Acadians than among the Anglophone population indicates that the cultural oppression of Acadians is reflected in the area of mental health. There is a further element of ethnic oppression in that the outlook of the specialist, who is usually Anglophone, carries with it a whole relationship of domination and exclusion of the Acadian minority. In this sense, the treatment process must necessarily exclude the different way of life that characterizes the Acadians. It is clear that the principle of "legitimate reality" is the reality of the majority. Frantz Fanon and Alfa Ibrahim Sow drew similar conclusions from studies carried out on other population groups.[11] York University sociologist John O'Neill's explanation of the racist nature of colonial medicine and psychology, citing Fanon, has already been noted (see page 38).

If the various groups had the same conception of what is socially unacceptable, the rate of involuntary admission could be expected to be the same. Because the difference in that rate is so pronounced, the hypothesis of repression of minority groups through psychiatry is a plausible one.

5.4 FAMILY SIZE AND INVOLUNTARY CONFINEMENT

Examination of the files shows a striking difference in numbers of children between Acadian families and families in the other groups. Closer analysis confirms this observation: for Loyalists confined to psychiatric institutions, the average number of children per family was 2.36; for the Irish, it was 2.43 per family; and for the Scots, it was 2.57. For the Acadians, it was almost double — 4.77 children per family on the average. The largest number of children found was sixteen. As one participant said, "a family like that is enough to drive a woman crazy."

Trying to verify whether these statistics were representative of the population as a whole proved to be a difficult task. Statistics Canada does not use the same criteria as the psychiatric institutions to calculate the number of children in a family. Statistics Canada brings in age, education and the number of marriages as variables and counts only children who are under twenty-one years of age and living at home. With the caveats imposed by these limitations, the following figures can be given: the average number of children per family in New Brunswick in 1961 and 1966 was 2.3, while in 1971 it fell to 2.0.[12] In Canada as a whole, families in the category of "English mother tongue" had an average of 2.45 children in 1971, while for "French mother tongue" families the Canadian average was 2.98.

Table 11
Percentage of Admissions That Are Involuntary by Sex and Marital Status, 1956-81

Group	Single Men	Women	Married Men	Women	Separated or Divorced Men	Women	Widowed Men & Women
English	67.8	68.0	42.9	60.9	73.7	40.0	Number
Acadian	69.0	65.3	65.6	74.6	77.8	50.0	too small

Using these Statistics Canada figures, the number of children per family for Acadians admitted to psychiatric institutions is higher than the average for Francophone families. However, for Anglophone families, the Statistics Canada average and the statistics for people admitted to psychiatric institutions are the same.

The relationship between number of children and the likelihood of being admitted involuntarily to a psychiatric institution is an area to be studied further. I have only raised the possibility of such a relationship here.

5.5 MULTIVARIATE ANALYSIS: INVOLUNTARY ADMISSION, SEX, ETHNIC ORIGIN AND MARITAL STATUS

We will continue the preceding analysis by combining the four variables we have examined. Because of the number of variables being cross-tabulated and the small number of Irish and Scottish subjects, the results for these two groups were omitted. The data in table 11 support our earlier comparisons of rates of involuntary admission on the basis of sex and ethnic origin. In both the English-speaking and Acadian groups, married women were admitted involuntarily much more often than married men. On the other hand, separated or divorced men were admitted involuntarily much more often than separated or divorced women.

5.6 METHOD OF ADMISSION AND OCCUPATION

In the study of confinement in the nineteenth century cited in chapter 2, individuals with no occupation were overrepresented in the institutions of the time. Interestingly, the same tendency can be seen today: 74.5 per cent of the case histories analysed for this study were those of "housewives" (22.7 per cent), "unemployed" (37.3 per cent) or "labourers" (14.5 per cent) admitted involuntarily.

Comparison of occupation and rate of involuntary admission shows that individuals in these three categories are confined involuntarily more often than others. It would seem that the more socially respected the occupation, the lower the rate of involuntary admission. In this respect, housewives and professionals are at totally opposite ends of the scale (figure 10).

Figure 10
Percentage of Admissions That Are
Involuntary by Occupation, 1956-81

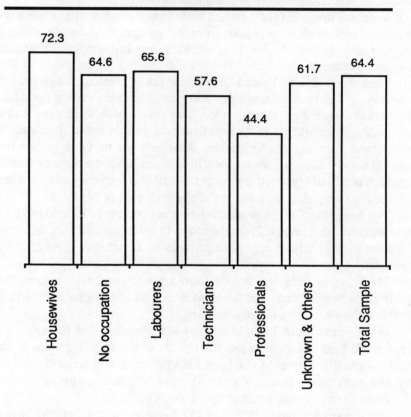

It should be noted that unemployment is much higher in Acadian areas. At the time this study was carried out, according to Statistics Canada, the unemployment rate was higher in the northeastern and northwestern parts of the province, where there are the highest concentrations of Francophones. This raises the possibility of a relationship between involuntary hospitalization and unemployment. According to our sample, three quarters of those admitted to psychiatric institutions are either largely or completely unintegrated into the "working world." Are such people excluded because they are considered nonproductive? Or does the fact of being unemployed create a predisposition to mental illness, as some recent studies seem to show?[13]

Acadians are constantly forced to follow a pattern that is alien and unnatural to them. If they deviate from this pattern, there are a number of ways of making them "normal" again, including involuntary hospitalization and treatment.

Most Acadians, and Acadian housewives in particular, fall into the category of "inferior social status," according to a study carried out during the period covered by this survey.[14] This refers both to income and to occupational mobility and its ramifications. In this sense, it is easy to understand Acadian out-migration. Acadians go to Ontario, western Canada and the United States to look for a better life and a more promising future. They will try anything to get out of the trap they are in which threatens to snap shut on them at the slightest sign of deviance.

Can being outside the productive process and the industrial model of development be a reason for involuntary hospitalization? Figure 10 and the following examples appear to provide an affirmative answer to this question:

Mr. X, aged forty-six, comes from a French-speaking region; "socially maladjusted, does not function well, considering he claims to be unable to work," notes his psychiatrist.

Mr. Z, from Saint John, is seventy-six. Here is what he says: "I'm depressed; I sit and think a lot, mainly about the fact that I am in this hospital and that I shouldn't be here; I have always worked hard, now I'm old and can't earn a living. My family have all passed away..."

Even in psychiatric institutions, work is valued.

Mr. V was admitted in 1939; in 1952, his report noted that "this patient does not talk, does not work in the room."

Is it a coincidence that he was still in Centracare in 1981?

Mr. T, admitted in 1936, during the Depression, was worried because he was unable to find work. A year later, his file noted that he was "not destructive or violent." However, in 1944, he was described as dirty and dangerous and had to be tied down constantly. In 1962, his situation had not improved, and he was put into a rehabilitation group. He was still in Centracare in 1981, after forty-two years of institutional treatment.

The individual in the following example was admitted against her will because she refused to work:

Mrs. X, from an industrial town, was sent to Centracare "because she won't wash and refuses to work." Five months later, she had received sixty-nine insulin shock treatments in fifty-five hours of treatment. Her psychiatrist's conclusion, noted in her file, was that "in fact, she hasn't made any progress; on the contrary, her condition has worsened."

Even the psychiatric hospital has to integrate its patients into the productive process, into the world of work. As Christian Delacampagne has written:

But the hospital, with its institutional inertia, resists, and will continue to resist for a long time. The eventual price will be that it will have to make a whole series of compromises with progressive critics. One of the major concessions it may have to make will be the introduction of work into the asylum, thus bringing the hospital more in line with life, or more precisely with the needs of the capitalist economy. Is there any method of rehabilitation better than work? And is there a surer way of exploiting — or, in other words, reintegrating into the system — those who, through their deviance, have tried to exclude themselves from that system? In short, delinquents, mad people, and even people suffering from tuberculosis can, through work, be both reeducated and reintegrated into the productive process, which is also a preventive process: a person who works can't do anything bad.[15]

Table 12
Percentage of Admissions That Are Involuntary by Occupation, Sex and Language, 1956-81

	Seasonal workers Men	House- wives Women	No occupation Men	No occupation Women	Technical workers Men
French	76.2	81.0	68.7	62.1	55.9
English	54.2	60.8	75.9	31.1	45.2

Note: Other categories were not included in this table because the samples were too

5.7 METHOD OF ADMISSION, OCCUPATION AND LANGUAGE

In order to determine whether the rate of involuntary admission varies according to ethnic group within the same occupational category, a few occupations were isolated for closer analysis. Given the small number of Irish and Scots, all the English-speaking groups were considered together.

Table 12 shows a marked difference among women in terms of mother tongue. Whether they were housewives or identified as having no occupation, Francophone women were admitted more frequently than Anglophone women. The difference between Anglophones and Francophones in the rate of involuntary admission was very high in women with no paid employment, fairly high (10 to 20 per cent) in men who were seasonal labourers and women who were housewives, and slight in the two other categories.

There was a very high rate of involuntary admission in men with no stated occupation, especially among Anglophones, while for women with no paid employment, the rate was very low.

This table, looked at together with other information presented earlier, indicates that a number of factors must be brought into play to explain involuntary admission to psychiatric institutions, the most significant up to this point being ethnic origin, marital status, occupation and possibly the number of children.

Table 13 confirms previous observations regarding marital status, language and sex. Here again, because the analysis uses four variables, the entire English-speaking sample has been grouped together under a single heading. In tables 12 and 13, three groups have disproportionately high rates of involuntary admission:

Table 13
Percentage of Admissions That Are Involuntary by Language and Marital Status, 1956-81

Sex and marital status	Language	%
Married men	English	46.7
	French	66.7
Married women	English	58.8
	French	75.8

• the unemployed or people who work in occupations society views as marginal (people with no occupation, housewives, seasonal workers).

• Acadians: in all categories except one (men with no occupation), the rate of involuntary admission is higher for Acadians than for English-speaking ethnic groups. As well, an individual who is both an Acadian and unemployed has a double handicap in terms of likelihood of being committed to an institution.

• married women: this shows up especially clearly in table 13.

5.8 DIAGNOSIS AND ETHNIC ORIGIN

Every file contains a preliminary diagnosis established when the patient undergoes a psychiatric examination on admission. This diagnosis can be changed a number of times during the patient's stay in hospital. This study takes into account only the diagnosis on the admission form, in other words, the first diagnosis in the file. An analysis of the diagnoses made for the three groups in our study appears in table 14. These results show:

• that Acadians were three times more likely than the "English" group, and seven times more likely than the Irish group, to have their psychiatric problems diagnosed as neurosis.

• that Acadians were diagnosed as psychotic and mentally deficient more often than the other groups.

Table 14
Diagnosis on Admission by Ethnic Group, 1956-81

| Diagnosis | % | | |
	English	Irish	Acadian
Neurosis	7.6	2.8	20.4
Psychosis	15.2	13.9	18.0
Schizophrenia	25.1	22.2	19.0
Alcoholism	21.8	38.9	12.3
Mental deficiency	4.7	5.6	8.8
Observation	2.4	0	1.4
Personality disorder	11.4	11.1	8.5
Affective disorder and depression	8.0	0	7.7
Others	3.8	5.5	3.9
Total	100	100	100

• that English-speaking people were diagnosed as schizophrenic more frequently than the other groups. Schizophrenia is considered a "modern-day" illness.

• that a very high percentage of Irish were admitted for alcoholism; it must be said that the Irish have a widespread reputation for their use of alcoholic beverages. It was said of the first Irish immigrants to the United States: "The indulgence of their appetites for stimulating drinks ... and their strong love for their native land ... are the fruitful causes of insanity among them. As a class, we are not so successful in our treatment of them as with the native population of New England. It is difficult to obtain their confidence, for they seem to be jealous of our motives."[16]

• that there is, on the other hand, less neurosis among the Irish, and much less alcoholism diagnosed in Acadians.

Analysis of table 14 indicates that there are very pronounced differences among the three groups in terms of the diagnoses made on admission. This would tend to confirm that the psychiatric institution is a means of excluding the socially unacceptable, and that it reflects the cultural norms imposed by the powerful in society on deviant individuals and minority groups.[17]

5.9 ADMISSION TO PSYCHIATRIC INSTITUTIONS AND PLACE OF RESIDENCE

An initial observation based on table 15 is that Saint John has the province's highest per capita rate of admission to psychiatric institutions. We can attribute this, as Riley and Richman do, to proximity to a psychiatric hospital.[18] Campbellton also has a psychiatric institution; the number of admissions per 100,000 inhabitants for that city is lower than for Saint John, but higher than for other areas.

For purposes of analysis, data on admissions to psychiatric institutions were compared to the total number of inhabitants for each locality, according to official Statistics Canada figures for 1981. In order to understand table 15, it should be noted that Saint John is the only city in New Brunswick that has experienced significant industrial development: it is a port city, has an oil refinery, and is also the headquarters of the Irving family empire, the largest concentration of industrial capital in the province. Many Acadians are obliged to work there because they are unable to find jobs elsewhere in New Brunswick. The unemployment rate is lower than the provincial average.

Table 15
Total Number of Admissions to Psychiatric Institutions
per 100,000 population, New Brunswick, 1956-81

Population category	1981 population	Admissions per 100,000 population
Saint John*	80,523	162
Campbellton*	9,818	115
Cities with more than 20,000 population	98,466	47
Cities and towns between 5,000 and 20,000 population	70,215	134
Rural areas (less than 5,000 population)	398,230	70

*Site of a psychiatric institution

Taking up the theory developed by the philosopher Paul Janet, Roger Bastide outlines the pressures that urbanization inflicts on individuals, and suggests that this factor plays a role in the process of exclusion and confinement:

So long as society does not create problems which are too difficult and does not demand too much of the individual, subjects who are disposed to psychic disorders can succeed in adapting and in leading a normal existence; this is what happens in homogeneous and traditional communities, such as rural communities. But in the progressive and heterogeneous modern city competition and the struggle for higher economic and social status lead us rapidly to burn up our last resources.[19]

According to table 15, there seems to be a relationship between proximity to psychiatric institutions and the rate of admission. Saint John and Campbellton have the highest rates of admission in the province. Saint John, as well as being the most highly industrialized city, also has the highest rate of involuntary admissions. However, on the basis of the evidence, it is impossible to say that the industrialization factor is necessarily more significant than the proximity factor in explaining these figures.

The other two cities with populations of over 20,000 are not highly industrialized like Saint John. The role of Fredericton, the provincial capital, is clearly much more political than industrial. Moncton, while highly developed in terms of both industry and services, is quite far away from the two psychiatric institutions, and, in its case, the proximity factor may work to keep the rate down.

What, then, is the situation of Acadians in Saint John? Might not the fact that they are living in an industrial city, forced to work and function in a strange, English-dominated milieu, be reflected in the rate of admission to psychiatric institutions?

According to Statistics Canada figures, 5,620 Acadians lived in Saint John in 1981; with an Anglophone population of 76,480, the Acadians represented 7.3 per cent of the total. According to our study, Acadians represent 21.9 per cent of admissions to psychiatric institutions from Saint John — exactly three times the percentage of Acadians in the city's overall population. In other words, an Acadian living in Saint John is three times more likely to be admitted to the local psychiatric institution than an Anglophone living in the same city. It should not be forgotten that Saint John already has the highest rate of admission in the province.

A similar analysis has been done for Campbellton. Anglophones, who are in the minority there, are involuntarily hospitalized more often than Francophones (150 per 100,000 inhabitants for Anglophones and 80 per 100,000 inhabitants for Francophones). This seems to indicate that members of a minority group, be it Anglophone or Francophone, are likely to be excluded much more often than members of the dominant group, which has appropriated the right to impose its way of life and punish those who do not fit in.

5.10 PORTRAIT OF A TYPICAL INVOLUNTARY INMATE OF A PSYCHIATRIC INSTITUTION

A number of factors can be used to interpret our data on involuntary hospitalization — geographic proximity to psychiatric institutions, culture shock, different values, distance from the traditional social milieu, displacement from ethnic roots, marital status. There are undoubtedly others, but these are the most significant in the context of this study.

A description of the oppression suffered by Acadians in industrialized society can be applied to the oppression all Acadians encounter just by living in a province where the prevailing values and the political context make them outsiders. This observation can help in interpreting the rate of involuntary admission among Acadians, which is much higher than the provincial average. As David Riesman has written, "these people have their choice, if indeed there be a choice, between homelessness and rapid acculturation to other-directed values."[20]

As well, it is apparent that both in the nineteenth century and today, the majority of involuntary inmates of psychiatric institutions have come from the lower socioeconomic echelons, and that most of those with paid employment work in menial jobs. More often, people who are admitted involuntarily are not even part of the official work force: they are unemployed, have no stated occupation or are housewives.

What conclusions can be drawn from this study of involuntary hospitalization? First of all, it is clear that in New Brunswick, mental health legislation is very often used to admit, against their will, people who are considered a danger to themselves or to others. At the beginning of this chapter, it was emphasized that the terms of the legislation lend themselves to a number of interpretations and therefore to abuse both by the population as a whole and by specialists responsible for involuntary admissions.

Assuming that involuntary admission is an act of oppression, we can conclude that the involuntary admission provisions of the Mental Health Act target certain sectors of the New Brunswick population more than others, and therefore that these sectors are more oppressed than others. They include Acadians as opposed to other ethnic groups, married women as opposed to unmarried women, and people with certain types of occupations, particularly those considered to have low social status. Finally, on the basis of the variables taken into account, certain categories appear to be more vulnerable when they have more than one "handicap": married housewives, Acadians living in Saint John, widowers.

In terms of diagnosis, the strikingly high percentage of neurosis among Acadians cannot go unmentioned. It must be asked whether this is not a tangible sign of the oppression suffered by Acadians both now and in the past.

Our statistical study confirms some of the findings of Durkheim and Fanon for the case of New Brunswick. Durkheim found that married women and unmarried men had a higher rate of suicide than unmarried women and married men. Our study of involuntary confinement leads us to the same results for these two variables. Fanon concluded, on the basis of his study of the situation in North Africa, that colonized and oppressed peoples suffer from disorders that psychiatry tries to attribute to individual causes. In this sense, in the way they are viewed and treated by psychiatry, Acadians resemble the African peoples colonized by Europe.

NOTES

1. See Marc-Adélard Tremblay and Gérald Louis Gold, *Communautés et culture: éléments pour une ethnologie du Canada français* (Montreal: HRW, 1973); Charles Hughes et al., *People of Cove and Woodlot* (New York: Basic Books, 1960); Robert Mayer and Henri Dorvil, "La Psychiatrie au Québec: réalité d'hier, pratique d'aujourd'hui," in Association Canadienne de Sociologie et d'Anthropologie de Langue Française, *Rapport du Colloque* (Montreal: Editions Saint-Martin, 1982), pp.111-29; Anne Paquet-Deehy et al., "Les femmes sont-elles plus malades que les hommes?", unpublished paper delivered in Halifax, June 1981; Néré St-Amand, "La Santé mentale au Nouveau-Brunswick, bref historique et observations," *Revue de l'Université de Moncton* 13, no. 3 (1980): pp.167 -85.

2. New Brunswick, Department of Health, *Annual Report* ; 1981.

3. Pierre Godin, *Cinq ans de trop* (Petit-Rocher, N.B., 1971), pp. 28, 34.

4. See Michel Roy, *L'Acadie perdue* (Montreal: Québec/Amérique, 1978).

5. Rodney Riley and Alex Richman, "Involuntary Hospitalization to Mental and Psychiatric Hospitals in Canada," unpublished paper delivered in Winnipeg, September 1981, p. 12.

6. See Tremblay and Gold, *Communautés et culture* .

7. Phyllis Chesler, *Women and Madness* (New York: Avon Books, 1973), p. 39.

8. See Jacques Donzelot, *The Policing of Families* (New York: Pantheon Books, 1979).

9. See Walter R. Gove and Jeannette F. Tudor, "Adult Sex Role and Mental Illness," *American Journal of Sociology* 78:812 - 35.

10. Paquet-Deehy et al., "Les femmes sont-elles?"

11. Frantz Fanon, *The Wretched of the Earth* (New York: Grove Press, 1966); Alfa Ibrahim Sow, *Anthropological Structures of Madness in Black Africa* (New York: International Universities Press, 1980).

12. Canada, Statistics Canada, Halifax Regional Office, conversation with the author; data for 1971.

13. See Sharon Kirsh, *Unemployment, Its Impact on Body and Soul* (Toronto: Canadian Mental Health Association, 1983).

14. Alain Even, "Le Territoire pilote du Nouveau-Brunswick ou les blocages culturels au développement économique," doctoral thesis, Faculté de droit et de Sciences économiques, Université de Rennes, 1970.

15. Christian Delacampagne, *Figures de l'oppression* (Paris: Presses Universitaires de France, 1977).

16. David Rothman, *The Discovery of the Asylum* (Boston: Little, Brown and Co., 1971), p. 284.

17. See Fanon, *Wretched of the Earth* ; R.D. Laing and David Cooper, *Reason and Violence: A Decade of Sartre's Philosophy* (London: Tavistock Publications, 1964).

18. Riley and Richman, "Involuntary Hospitalization."

19. Roger Bastide, *The Sociology of Mental Disorder* (London: Routledge and Kegan Paul, 1972), p. 18.

20. David Riesman, *The Lonely Crowd* (New Haven: Yale University Press, 1961), p. 35.

6

How New Brunswickers Look at Madness

If you talk about Emerie LeBlanc, they won't know who you're talking about; but if you talk about Emerie Fou, then they'll know.

It so happened that he was getting paid for being crazy...
— *from interviews with Acadians*

6.1 METHODOLOGY

In the following pages, interviews with Acadian, Irish and Loyalist New Brunswickers living in a variety of settings are analysed. Working from the hypothesis that individuals express their conditions of existence in their own speech, I asked at least eight people in each group about their ideas of mental illness, madness and exclusion. These interviews averaged twenty-five pages in length. They were analysed by decoding them to identify the signs of representation of objective reality in the discourse.

Subjects living in an industrialized setting were chosen from the population of Moncton, New Brunswick's second largest industrial city. According to Statistics Canada, Moncton had a population of 55,000 in 1981. It is also the railway capital of the Maritime provinces. I was able to interview four people of Acadian descent, six of Irish origin and four Loyalists.

It was learned from a preliminary enquiry that there was a significant concentration of people of Irish descent in Melrose, a community of about three hundred people some seventy kilometres from Moncton, and so rural Irish were chosen from this community. Melrose was founded more than a century ago by a group of immigrants who came directly from Ireland, and was a thriving agricultural centre until the 1950s. Since then, young people have gradually left Melrose, and both its population and its economy have been in decline. Now people pass through Melrose on their way to get the ferry to Prince Edward Island. Four interviews were conducted there.

The rural Acadian community chosen was Cap-Pelé, a fishing village about fifty kilometres from Moncton whose population is more than 95 per cent Acadian. Six interviews suitable for analysis were conducted in Cap-Pelé.

Finally, Salisbury was chosen as a rural community with a large number of people of Loyalist descent.* It has a population of almost 1,700 and is about forty kilometres from Moncton. The leading occupations in Salisbury are agriculture and fur farming. Here, four interviews could be used for analysis, while a fifth person refused to be taped.

Content analysis by semantic field was the primary method used to analyse these interviews. A picture of what is considered abnormal, from the person who needs a little extra attention to the deviant for whom institutionalization is regarded as the only solution, emerged from words that recurred frequently in the participants' discourse. The words with the highest frequency of occurrence were highlighted for purposes of analysis.

Content analysis was used because it allows the researcher to draw conclusions about the subject under study on the basis of indicators. As Laurence Bardin has written:

The content analyst is like an archaeologist. He works from traces — the "documents" he is able to find or elicit. But these traces are manifestations of states, data, phenomena. Through them and thanks to them, something can be discovered. Just as ethnography needs ethnology to interpret its detailed descriptions, the operations that the content analyst performs on the messages he deals with take the form of logical deductions that bear fruit as conclusions about the author of the message or his environment, for example.[1]

This aspect of the research was aimed at establishing "a correspondence between semantic or linguistic structures and psychological or sociological structures."[2] The method consisted of first identifying all the occasions where particular words were used and then grouping them by theme to make it possible to draw conclusions.

The first step was a preliminary reading of the transcripts to identify words and expressions referring to the semantic field of madness that were used frequently by the participants (a total of at least five occurrences in the interviews with members of a particular ethnic group). A list of words in each language was drawn up. No correspondence between words was assumed at the outset; thus, *fou* and *crazy* were not necessarily considered synonyms. In this way, a collection of terms referring directly to the semantic field of madness was identified for each of the three groups. It

---

*Salisbury would be the subject of national attention in August 1987 when residents protested the appointment of a Francophone from northern New Brunswick as the town's postmaster.

was also possible to conclude from this preliminary reading that the participants often referred to care and the care system for the mentally ill, so that the following terms were also brought into the analysis: *soin*, *soigner*, *aide*, *traiter* and *traitement* in French, and *care*, *help*, *treat* and *treatment* in English.

The sentences containing words regarded as having significance were set aside. These segments taken from the interviews were then classified according to whether the speaker was an urban or rural resident and which ethnic group he or she belonged to. Then, each of the terms chosen for study was analysed in detail to determine what the word signified in its immediate context and what general orientation emerged from looking at all these words for a particular ethnic group. The results of this research are presented separately for each ethnic group. Then, the three groups are compared in an effort to establish similarities and differences in terms of the analysis as a whole.

6.2 HOW ACADIANS EXPLAIN MADNESS

6.2.1 The Process of Medicalization: From Care to Treatment

"Medicalization" is used here to describe a greater hold over society by medical power through medicine and its institutions. Medical power penetrates the social fabric, as Michel Foucault said, and by enforcing its norms becomes one of the instruments by which old beliefs and traditions are broken down and Acadians become part of industrial society. New Brunswick's equal opportunity program in the 1960s involved this form of subjugation: economic and political integration took place through the state's ideological apparatus in general and through the health and education systems in particular.

The concepts of *"soin"* (care) and *"aide"* (help)

We will first look at the words *care* and *help* , which are related to the rest of the analysis and useful in clarifying its significance.

Both these words involve a need that the individual cannot fulfill on his or her own, and generally refer to daily life. They imply that the individual has recourse to another person for some form of assistance. In the case of *care*, this other person is often a doctor; in fact, a doctor was mentioned explicitly in four of ten references. By contrast, the concept of *help* refers more to local and community support systems. In one case, "the priest" and "the hospital" were referred to; in another case, simply "a person." In other instances, even though no particular group or individual was referred to, the implication was that help was provided by a nonprofessional.

On two occasions both concepts, *care* and *help*, appeared in the same sentence; this is why they were grouped together. It is, in any case, easy to see clear links between the two: both refer to a need that is felt when daily life becomes threatening:

The care they need.

He really needs care.

A relationship with work was mentioned several times:

Work was hard, it made me tired, there was no way I could stay home to take care of myself.

This appears to suggest that *care-help* is incompatible with work. A person who can no longer function productively in daily life needs *help* or *care.*

Since the 1960s, the Acadian people and their elite have been demanding that therapeutic services be distributed more equitably by language group. They want more medical and psychiatric services. Following David Riesman's analysis, the idea of *help* refers to a traditional way of life and societal network. *Care*, on the other hand, implies a professional and an institutional network of services, and would refer more to an inner-directed social model, involving a gradual break with family and friends and greater recourse to a professional who is a stranger to the immediate social context.

In addition, both these words imply a support system outside the institution: where possible, help and care are provided; if these approaches don't work, you resort to the institution. Acadians appear to favour the traditional network of responsibility for health. This would mean that the Acadian community maintains a degree of autonomy and independence with respect to the institutional network, which is more highly developed in urban settings.

It is worth noting that one participant clearly dissociated *care* from the institution. One had a local, community connotation, while the other involved keeping watch rather than taking care:

Now if she wanted to kill herself or something like that, if a person couldn't watch over her all the time, I suppose you would have to send her somewhere where she could be watched over, you know, because in cases like that, you can take care of them for a while, but there comes a time when you get tired, you would become just like her. ...

This interview gives some indication of Acadians' tolerance for mental illness: *help* and *care* constitute a response to attitudes and behaviours that are different but acceptable. By contrast, a more pronounced difference quickly becomes labelled, and the person is locked into a status of marginality and deviance. It seems paradoxical, however, that these people know that they are sending their sick loved ones to psychiatric institutions to be sheltered and watched over. Are they trying to salve their consciences, knowing full well that the institution is not part of the network of "helping" and "caring"?

The terms *"traiter"* (treat) and *"traitement"* (treatment)

These two terms are presented together for purposes of analysis. Unlike *care* and *help*, they imply that the individual does not participate in his or her rehabilitation.

It seems to me that they said once that there was somebody who gave treatments. ...

In none of the interviews was an individual who underwent *treatment* described as participating actively in the management of his or her own case. Instead, this responsibility was entrusted to an expert — in this case a psychiatrist — and the institution.

He saw the whole treatment that took place there [in the psychiatric hospital].

They [the psychiatrists in Saint John] treated her and then she got better after a while.

The term *treatment* is also used specifically to designate electroconvulsive therapy: a number of participants used the English expression *shock treatment* . The participants had no trouble justifying this form of intervention when the individual's situation went beyond certain limits:

There have to be treatments. There have to be places for those people.

Another person gave an idea of the threshold for using this form of therapy — when what is happening is no longer understood:

Well, she had a case of nerves, she was screaming, crying, you couldn't understand what was wrong. That's what they did, they treated her and then she got better after a while.

This quotation suggests the beneficial results of "treatment." By contrast, another interview gave the impression that treatments didn't help — quite the reverse, in fact:

There was a case, a young guy here, not far from here, and I think he went for treatments. When he was three or four years old, he could read

French and English. He was quite intelligent, and then, he was twenty-four or twenty-five I think, and then he became so intelligent that he went over the top, and it's like he became a child again, you know.

Although the participants gave no precise definition of what treatment involves, it can be concluded that treatment typically takes place inside rather than outside the institution and that psychiatrists in particular assume responsibility for it.

6.2.2 Terms the Acadians Use to Describe Mental Illness

The words and expressions that occurred most often in the interviews are presented here in ascending order from those designating conditions regarded as the most benign and tolerable to those designating conditions considered the most dangerous.

The term *"retardé"* (retarded)

This term, frequently used in French Canada, is borrowed from the English phrase *mentally retarded.*

A person designated by this term in the interviews was always characterized by a congenital condition. Nevertheless, some progress is possible because these people can learn:

They are intelligent in their fashion.

You can make them do things. It seems they can make progress.

However, no intrinsic change seems to be possible:

They are not going to change.

These individuals are different from others but they are not dangerous, and in this sense, the community can adapt to them and accept them:

At that time, someone who was born retarded, they used to keep him.

An analysis of the interviews indicates the needs of this group: care, attention and special schools. The concept of *retarded* was used ten times, and in five of these cases the word *school* was associated with it. This suggests the idea of apprenticeship and possible progress, but not in a mainstream school environment. Retarded people are marginal in terms of their schooling, and as a result they have limited opportunities for socialization.

In sum, *mentally retarded* implies a degree of marginalization applying especially to children, refers to a congenital condition, and is apparently tolerated by the Acadian community, at least according to the interviews under study here. One participant mentioned the fact that retardation could lead to madness "if something happened":

If he went off, if something happened and he went mad, then they would have him examined by a doctor, the doctor would sign for him and they would sign to have him sent to Saint John to the "bug house"* as they called it.

The term *"pas normal"* (not normal)

This term is used in reference to something visible, something tangible: actions, words, incidents where the person is "sort of strange, lost." An element of danger also sometimes enters the picture:

I mean they would be doing something that is not normal to do; it could be serious or not so serious; if it's something dangerous, it wouldn't be good for them to stay home....

However, "not normal" people are dangerous only if they are associated with those who are "troubled" or "out of their minds." The needs of such people were referred to only once. In this case, they had to be sent to an institution when they were "afraid and lost." The expression *vraiment pas normal* (really not normal) was used in this case, indicating a turning point in the development of the pathology.

Participants associated this term with *écarté* (absent) and *perdu* (lost), suggesting a behaviour and a deviance that can be easily noticed. There are concrete signs so that a "not normal" person can be easily spotted by behaviour, speech or manner.

The word *"mental"* (mental)

The first recorded use of the word *mental* in French was in a work by J. de Vignay in 1327. The word is derived from the Latin *mens,* referring to the mind as a whole. In French, however, it very quickly took on an intellectual and normative, as opposed to affective, connotation. Thus, it refers to the capacity for learning, obeying laws, adapting to social values and taking responsibility for one's actions.

In Acadian speech, the expression *il est mental* (he is mental) or *il est devenu mental* (he has become mental) signifies that the person in question is unable to reason and adjust his or her behaviour to established norms. A person who has heavy equipment come to his house to take away the soil

---

*The term "bug house" is used both by English-speaking New Brunswickers, especially in the Saint John region, and by Acadians to designate an insane asylum.

to a depth of one metre because he says it's "magnetic" is described as "mental." So is someone who decides to go outside completely naked to wash himself in a barrel of water.

The word *mental* can also be an abbreviation for the expression *mentally ill* or *mental illness*. It designates an inability to get hold of oneself and take full responsibility for one's actions. A person who is mental, while not considered sick, "can't think", "imagines things," and "seems easily recognizable by sight." In general, a mental person is born mental, at least according to the expressions "I *am* not mental" and *"really* mental illnesses."* On the other hand, among the causes noted for this state are jealousy, drinking to excess, and a depression that was not properly cared for. This would indicate that one can also become "mental." Thus, a person is born mental or becomes mental, depending on the circumstances.

Mental is a synonym for *détraqué* (unhinged) or *manque de quoi dans la tête* (missing something in the head). It is clearly distinguished from *j'ai mon idée* (I can think), and hence characterizes people whose reason, whose mind, is not working properly. This suggests the importance of reason, of the mind as a logical instrument. People are "mental" when they do not have or are not in control of their intellectual capacities.

These people need institutional care, either in a psychiatric hospital or in a special home. Thus, the diagnosis of "mental" is a serious one and the traditional help-care network cannot meet the needs of this category.

It is noteworthy that two participants used the term *mental* to refer to the institution, a usage that is not common in French. One used the phrase *école mentale* (mental school) while the other referred to the *hôpital mental* (mental hospital). Several experts were consulted to help explain this construction. The following were considered possible interpretations:

• The participants could simply mean "an institution for the mentally ill," a phrase that they would abbreviate for practical reasons.

• The Acadians could be literally translating the English terms *mental hospital* and *mental place*, which are common informal substitutes for *psychiatric hospital* and *psychiatric institution*.

• The association of *mental* with *institution* could also be related to the above comments about the institution that does not care or help but keeps people for a long time. It would crystallize a conception of the institution and sum up the image that people have of it. According to this interpretation, a mental person would be sent to the mental institution, so that madness and the mad person would be on the same ground.

The term *"déprimé"* (depressed)

The words *dépression, depressed** and *déprimé* have been linked together for purposes of analysis because of their common semantic root. In general, they refer to more or less benign situations where what is required is the help of a friend.

People who are "just depressed" should see someone who loves them, rather than leaving for...

However, when the expression *really depressed* is used, the situation appears more serious and requires care rather than help. According to one participant, depression can lead to a more serious mental condition:

If it's not cared for right away, it can lead to really mental illnesses later on.

In this sense, depression can be interpreted as a forerunner, a predisposition, a warning.

A "depressed" person is regarded as "not too normal" and as suffering from an ill-defined malaise. In the case of a "not normal" person, on the other hand, there are clear signs. Depression is an internal, almost mysterious state:

I could never describe it because I couldn't see what she had, what she felt ... I believed it when she told me ... I mean, I don't know what she had ...

The term *"dérangé"* (disturbed)

This term is somewhat vague, and is often used to designate a series of inexplicable acts, "a bunch of things that you don't know what it is." A disturbed person "doesn't have good sense," or "can't learn." In other words, a disturbed person can do things that we wouldn't do. Disturbed people can nevertheless continue to work, although they are liable to be teased on the job more than other people:

When they see the slightest sign that a guy is a little disturbed, they'll start to pick on him.

This same participant also suggested that a disturbed person doesn't do the same kind of work as other people:

He didn't have a job like the others, his work was sweeping the place, picking up the dirt and so on ...

Whether or not disturbed people are integrated into the work world,

* This and other English terms are sometimes used by Acadians.

whether or not they carry their weight and contribute to society constitutes an important factor in the degree to which these people are accepted. In sum, limits are recognized, but the contribution — the economic usefulness — of the disturbed person is accepted.

In the interviews, *disturbed* was associated with *chaviré* (upset) and clearly distinguished from *normal* and *smart* . A whole range of possible needs for the disturbed person was suggested, from the help of the priest and the need for quiet, through hospitalization when a person is "so disturbed," to confinement in a psychiatric institution. In this last case, however, people's perception of the institution is not entirely positive:

Then they took her to Saint John, but they didn't keep her and then they said they couldn't do anything for her there.

A person is not sent to an institution simply as a result of being "disturbed." The person must also have done something that is considered serious, and it appears to be this act that sets off the process of confinement. Thus, being "disturbed" is not considered serious in itself, but some things that a disturbed person does could be threatening to the social order.

One participant mentioned that the priest should be consulted before a disturbed person is referred to the medical system. This was a common procedure among Acadians, and reflected a traditional conception of health services. Before calling in a health professional, Acadians consulted their parish priest, and generally followed his advice. If the priest recommended a medical or psychiatric assessment, they tended to respect his opinion. One psychiatrist noted that in 1982 he warned a priest to "stick to his crucifix and his church, and not to play the expert in psychiatry." He concluded: "Let each person stay on his own turf."

The following quotation illustrates the change from the traditional to the institutional care network in Acadia. The priest serves as an intermediary between the two systems:

One night, the mother called [the priest] because her daughter was so disturbed, to see if someone could go help her. The priest came, as he should, and tried to calm her, but the best thing was to have the ambulance come take her to the hospital. That was what they did. *

Whether or not "disturbed" people are accepted in their environment depends on their behaviour and their actions. A person whose actions are

---

*In all the interviews studied, this is the only reference to the clergy. This raises questions as to what the real role of the clergy is, both among Acadians and in the other two groups. This reference comes from an Acadian couple who live in a presbytery and whose job is to maintain the premises and cook for the resident priest.

socially useful may be laughed at and teased, but not excluded by being sent to an institution. On the other hand, people who commit dangerous acts are liable to confinement by virtue of their transgression against social norms. In talking about disturbed people, one participant raised the possibility that the norm may be subjective:

We're used to doing normal things — I mean in our heads they're normal; but for the others, the disturbed ones, maybe what they do is normal.

The expression *"sur les nerfs"* (a case of nerves)

The expressions *avec ses nerfs* and *sur les nerfs* (having a case of nerves), along with *nerveux* (nervous) and *maladie des nerfs* (nervous disease) have been grouped together under this heading.

In general, this situation is characterized by excess and lack of control. People who have a case of nerves are spoken of as being violent, destroying everything, shouting, crying, becoming malicious and dangerous. It is both an illness and a weakness. The participants believe that "nervous" people can be cured, and there is a whole range of possible treatments for them: drugs to calm them, home care, and, finally, confinement in the institution. In this sense, treatment is dissociated from the institution, which serves the purpose of control rather than treatment:

Those people have to be watched, they can be nasty, you know, and being nasty is dangerous. There are people who can be dangerous when they have a case of nerves.

Elsewhere, however, the same participant juxtaposed the institution with treatment:

It's a nervous disease, you know, it's nerves that cause a person to become like that, too disturbed; after that, nothing can be done with them. There have to be treatments. There have to be places for those people.

Causes mentioned were family, marital and work tensions, and a bad experience in religious life. It can be concluded that this is an acquired rather than a congenital phenomenon. *A case of nerves* is associated with being *disturbed* and with *madness*. It is clearly distinguished from *bons nerfs* (good nerves), which characterize a person who is smart and able to deal with and care for nervous people. One participant mentioned that a person with a nervous disease could be fired from his job, not because of the condition as such but because of actions that resulted from it:

He wasn't well, he had a nervous disease, then he was fired from Canadian National because he was fooling around. He wasn't doing his work the way he should ...

It is noteworthy that most of the causes associated with the problem of nerves are social: family tensions, difficulties at work, and noise were among the causes mentioned for nervous diseases. The situation becomes uncontrollable: the subject is no longer in control of his or her nervous system. Instead, nerves make the subject act; a kind of irrational force takes over the person and directs his or her actions.

As in the case of the disturbed person, the question of the economic usefulness of the person with a case of nerves was raised. If the person cannot work or is a source of amusement to others, this seems to be a litmus test, a criterion by which to judge the seriousness of his or her state. A person who fails this test represents a danger that threatens the system of production — as in the case of the individual who worked for the railway.

The expression *"perd la tête"* (out of one's mind)

The terms *perd la tête* and *hors de sa tête* (out of one's mind) are included under this heading. In general, these expressions are used to refer to people who have lost their reason. Two signs associated with this state are that a person "lost her memory" or "talks to himself." People who are out of their minds can also be dangerous:

Someone who's out of his mind, then all of a sudden, he gets it into his head to get his gun and then go shoot it.

Such people need to be cared for or else institutionalized, depending on the seriousness of their condition. Causes mentioned include drink, age and lack of sleep: "They said, well, he went to bed and fell asleep, he'll be better." Here too, the causes are not of a psychiatric nature, according to the participants. These expressions refer to a passing, temporary condition that can be cured through the traditional care system, except in the case of people who become dangerous, as noted above, or those whom the community wants to get rid of:

Then they decided they had no place to go; their relatives wouldn't bother with them so they decided to send them there [the institution].

People in the categories of *not normal, a case of nerves* and *out of their minds* are considered more dangerous than those in the categories of *mental, depressed* and *disturbed* (see figure 12, p. 118). And while this latter group of terms does not express any direct relationship with madness, the expressions *out of one's mind* and *a case of nerves* are associated with madness, with *can't reason* and *deranged* (see figure 11, p. 116). On the other hand, *not normal* is closer to *écarté* (absent) and *perdu* (lost). Finally, one participant implied that the institution could cause people to "go out of their minds":

Since she's been in the hospital, it's like she's out of her mind.

The word *"fou"* (mad, crazy)

This term occurred more frequently in the ten interviews with Acadians than any of the other terms studied — sixty-seven times. In addition, a number of participants hesitated to use the word, sometimes substituting a vague word or expression. In general, *fou* refers to someone who was born that way; sometimes, the word is even incorporated into the person's name:

You had to say Joe Fou, then you knew right away who that person was.

Another participant confirmed this observation, and went on to describe some of the things the person in question would do:

People call him the Fou, that's what his name is. It's how they christened him here. Now, he could be here where there are three forks in the road, eh, he could be in the middle, and if he wanted to piss, he would piss, that guy. He wouldn't wait to go to the bathroom, not him. I mean, a normal man wouldn't do something like that, as far as I know.

For disadvantaged people, the state of being crazy entails the financial advantage of being eligible for government assistance: "It so happened that he was getting paid for being crazy, but he wasn't the one getting paid, it was his relatives."* Thus, according to this observation, there may be an advantage in being crazy, but the individual doesn't necessarily benefit from it.

A person suffering from madness "can't earn a living", "isn't too smart," and is often "agitated." Some participants also indicated that they were afraid of crazy people, which meant that they often had to be locked up.

There were people who became like that, sort of crazy, as they say. They were dangerous, maybe they wanted to kill somebody, that was their whole idea: to take a gun and fire it.

There is a clear element of danger associated with this category: crazy people are a threat, by their condition if not by their actions. Seven causes were mentioned as being capable of bringing on madness: marital conflict,

---

* The original French is: "Ça fait que lui halait une paye de fou, mais c'est pas lui qui a la paye, c'est ses parents."

drugs, being driven crazy or taken for crazy by relatives, lack of sleep, alcohol abuse, and, according to one participant, even an overly difficult winter:

*During the winter, there was a family...they were troubled almost every winter...and they didn't sleep any more, and they became really crazy.**

It should be noted that none of the causes mentioned are strictly medical ones. These interpretations are different from the ones in psychiatry textbooks, where greater importance is given to psychological causes than to social and environmental factors.

Participants made a distinction between two categories of crazy people. The first consists of those whose condition is congenital; in this case, the nickname *fou* is attached to the person's given name, and *crazy* can be associated with *mental*. In the other category are people who have become crazy as a result of circumstances in their lives. In this case, *crazy* can be associated with *out of one's mind, nervous disease* and *se troubler* (troubled). In both cases, participants' interpretation of the cause of the condition differs from that of the experts, who concentrate more on internal, individual causes.

Crazy people are officially recognized as such — the government even pays them for being crazy, confirming the recognition and making it permanent. There is social recognition as well, as crazy people are easy to distinguish. They laugh for no reason, talk to themselves, are agitated — in short, they do irrational things. Crazy people are also described as being *pas très rusés* (not very smart). The fact that crazy people are unable to work completes the picture. And finally, others are afraid of them: they represent danger, not necessarily because of what they do but because of what they are believed to be capable of doing:

Other people would make him angry, they'd call him names, they'd call him all sorts of things, and then it happened that he was crazy, and he was nasty, he would swear, he would curse.

It is not hard to guess what sort of care is recommended for this category: they need to be watched over and confined. This tacitly suggests the incurable nature of their condition: in other words, to be crazy is to live the life of a social outcast:

He was a poor devil who picked up scraps here and there. ...

---

* The participant is referring to a family living in a remote area in the 1940s. During the winter months, the family was completely isolated from the rest of society.

The words *"trouble"* and *"troublé"* (troubled)

The "troubled" person is someone violent, someone who tries to escape, someone whose ideas make no sense and who could try to commit suicide. *Troubled* was twice associated with *crazy*; it is the opposite of *normal* and *smart*. Another participant described the troubled person as being "really crazy." Two levels of need were mentioned for this category: the institution and treatment. Neither care nor help is part of the therapy for troubled people. Even though this is not a congenital condition, the chance of rehabilitation appears to be slim:

When they' re troubled, people here, you can' t cure them, I don' t think.

Being troubled, like being crazy, is brought on by causes that are external to the individual and have to do with events in daily life: hard times, marital conflict, an overly long winter, poor fishing. These events in daily life, which can make a person "troubled," represent circumstances that the individual cannot easily control (the weather, fishing) or an unacceptable situation. The interviews suggest that we should look back at the concept of *trouble* in its wider sense, including its emotional and mental aspect.

The "troubled" person appears to reflect the collectivity's malaise and anguish, just as the Identified Patient in Virginia Satir's schema suffers the repercussions of a tense family situation. When this schema is transposed from the family to the social system, the "troubled" person takes the place of the Identified Patient, who serves both to crystallize tensions and to avoid them. The troubled person is thus the reflection and the proof of a troubled society that can acknowledge its troubles only through its deviants.[3]

Troubled people are betrayed by their actions — violence, homicide, suicide — and so it is easy to point one's finger at them: "You can see them by what they do, it's there for the whole world to see..."

The fact that Acadians have lived in a situation of constant oppression can make people troubled: "He was a man who was troubled, at that time, those people, they went through a lot of trouble to live." This interview raises the possibility that Acadians' historical and political situation could affect some individuals to the point of making them troubled.

On the basis of the danger they represent and the kind of treatment suggested for them, troubled people represent the most serious manifestation of madness in Acadians' eyes. This form of deviance is presented as both an individual and a social problem, at least in terms of its causes. Such people constitute a threat to the established order, because there appears — at least potentially — to be no bounds to what they might do. They also reflect an untenable social situation, in which even extreme solutions are considered. In this respect, their condition is analogous to anomie; in Durkheim's view, suicide could not be explained by individual causes alone. In his study, and in this one, the social context is a contributing factor as well.

6.2.3 Conclusion

In the preceding section, the significant terms used by Acadians in relation to mental illness were presented. These terms are useful in making clear how psychiatrically-based deviance can be interpreted socially.

For some people, the primary need is *care* and *help*; these are mostly people who fall into the categories of *retarded, depressed, disturbed, a case of nerves*, and *out of their minds*. For the last three of these conditions, the institution is also mentioned as a possibility when the traditional system of care is not successful. By contrast, care and help are not suggested for *crazy* and *troubled* people. Instead, such people need to be institutionalized, watched over and "treated" — a term that is not clearly defined. Thus, for some categories, the solution is removed from the *help-care* system and given over to the institution and "treatment," which represents the only recourse for the most serious or dangerous cases.

With the terms *a case of nerves, out of one's mind, troubled* and *crazy*; there are specific references to an element of danger. This would cast light on why people would want to put such individuals into the psychiatric institution. It is noteworthy that the causes cited to explain these conditions are neither medical nor psychiatric in nature.

The three concepts *a case of nerves, out of one's mind* and *troubled* are constantly associated with madness (being *crazy*) and vice versa. The schema (figure 11) shows the major poles of attraction linking the various terms. Pole A centres on the concept of madness and the institutional system as the solution people look towards, while pole B centres on a more socially acceptable form of abnormality, in which *disturbed* is the key term. The Acadian participants' conception of mental illness and the characteristics of the various categories noted in this chapter are presented in schematic form in figure 12 (p. 118). Showing the links among these categories represents an extension of this schematization.

Figure 11
Association Among Various Terms Used
by Acadians to Describe Madness

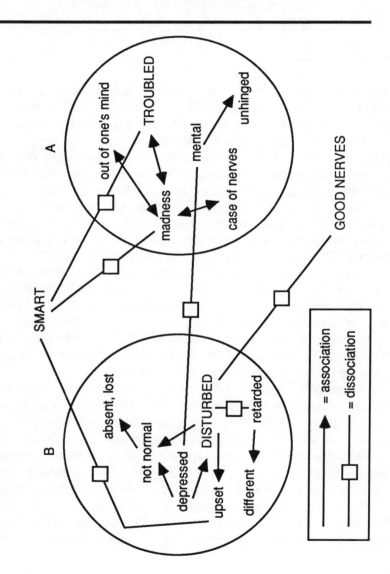

6.2.4 Trouble in Acadia

The results of this analysis show that the words *trouble* and *troubled* are significant for Acadians. The interviews indicate that people in this category are rejected primarily because of the danger they represent. Now that we have completed the descriptive stage of the content analysis, it is worth taking a closer look at the factors that explain the concepts we have examined, and especially the concept of *trouble*. Is there any basis for comparison between the psychiatric significance of this term and its current usage in Acadia? There are at least two possible interpretations.

(a) The political history of the Acadians and the events through which they have lived may constitute at least a partial explanation of both the social and the psychiatric meaning of trouble.

The following remarks are beyond the scope of the analysis as such, but they suggest an examination in greater depth of an element of the language that has come to the surface through the analysis.

An important characteristic of the *bon-ententisme* between Anglophones and Francophones in New Brunswick described earlier (see chapter 1) is that it implies the absence of *trouble* — of confrontation between the two language groups. In the interviews, there is an association between trouble and danger; the phenomena that cause this situation are external to the individual and often social in nature. Is it possible that the *fauteur de trouble* (troublemaker) is excluded because he or she constitutes a threat to the prevailing *bon-ententisme* and shows up its contradictions? It is not surprising that the powers and the elite associated with the established order would consider such a person dangerous and get rid of that person. Thus, the doctor and the psychiatrist would play a political and ideological role more than a medical one. The behaviour of the *fou*, the crazy person, is quite conventional, if not acceptable. The *fou* does not inspire fear and is easily labelled. By contrast, the behaviour of the *troubled* person is unpredictable and threatening. The condition is an acquired and hence contagious one. The *troubled* person *troubles* — in the primary sense of the word — the precarious Acadian equilibrium. In this context, it is worth recalling some recent "troubles" in Acadia and looking at the way the people responsible for the social agitation in question were integrated or excluded:

• 1968: crisis at the Université de Moncton; sociology department dismantled.

• 1970: beginning of controversy over Kouchibouguac National Park; events surrounding the "troublemaker" Jackie Vautour.

Figure 12
Acadians' Conception of Marginality and Deviance

Term	Congenital or Acquired	Requirements	Danger to Self or Others*	Associated with	Dissociated from	Special Features
Retarded	Congenital	• Care • Attention • School (apprenticeship)	-2	• Different	• Disturbed	• Associated with children • Marginal but acceptable
Mental	Congenital	• Institution	0	• Unhinged	• Able to think	• Applied by extension to the institution
Depressed	Congenital	• Help • Care	0	• Not too normal	• Real mental illnesses	•Less serious condition
Disturbed	Congenital	• Help • Institution	0	• Upset	• Normal • "smart"	• Can partici-pate in labour market
Not normal	Congenital and/or Acquired	• Control • Institution	+1	• Absent • Lost		• Related to behaviour, external signs
A case of nerves	Acquired	• Care • Institution	+2 -1	• Disturbed • Crazy	• Good nerves	• Causes relate to daily life
Out of one's mind	Acquired	• Care • Institution	+1	• Crazy • Can't reason		
Mad, crazy	Congenital and/or Acquired	• Observation • Confinement	+1 -1	• Out of one's mind • Nervous disease • Troubled		• All 6 causes relate to daily life • Can't work • Defined by actions
Troubled	Acquired	• Institution • Treatment	+3	• Crazy (twice) • Really crazy	• Smart • Normal	• Causes are social

* Figures indicate numbers of participants expressing the view that the category in question does or does not represent danger. Thus -2 indicates that two participants thought that "retarded" people are not dangerous; +1 indicates that one participant clearly expressed the view that "not normal" people are dangerous.

• 1970: beginning of attempt to organize the Maritime Fishermen's Union.

• 1975: beginning of crisis at Cirtex, Caraquet; elimination of the existing union.

• 1979: funds for the Société des Acadiens du Nouveau-Brunswick are cut drastically after the organization holds its national policy conference.

• 1981: students occupy the Université de Moncton; some are expelled for having taken part in the occupation; those who are readmitted are temporarily denied the right of association.

• Crisis at *L'Evangéline* ; sudden and permanent closure of the only Acadian daily newspaper after certain union demands are made.

Whether trouble is individual or collective, it involves a danger to the established order. Attempts are made to eliminate this trouble by identifying and marginalizing those responsible for it, finding victims, and intimidating the rest of the population. The transposition of the term *trouble* from the psychological to the political sphere clearly merits special attention in future research.

(b) Another possible explanation, again raised here in an exploratory fashion, is that for a people whose main occupation is fishing, trouble may suggest storms — a familiar image to seafarers. Expressions such as *la mer se trouble* (the sea is troubled), *l'eau est troublée* (the water is troubled), and *ce vent annonce du trouble* (this wind means trouble) are heard in common Acadian speech. Here too, trouble suggests a kind of bad omen, a difficult situation that becomes uncontrollable. To note just one example, 145 fishermen from the Acadian village of Baie Sainte-Anne were lost during a violent storm in 1959. A storm — a "troubled" sea — can have serious consequences.

These two interpretations are, of course, not necessarily mutually exclusive.

6.3 RESULTS OF INTERVIEWS WITH THE IRISH

As noted in chapter 1, the particular characteristic of the Irish is that they straddle the strict language-religion division represented by the other two target groups in this study. The Irish are generally Catholics like the Acadians, but speak English like the Loyalists. The interviews with Irish participants suggest three major headings. First, the various conceptions of mental illness held by the participants are outlined. The kinds of therapy the participants suggested constitute the second heading. And finally, the different forms that mental illness can take are examined. Note that this schema differs from the one used for the Acadians: this is because the Irish participants' concept of illness fits into a medical structure that concentrates more on symptoms and forms of treatment than on causes.

6.3.1 Conceptions of Illness

The concepts *"sick"* and *"sickness"*

In our discussion of the Acadians, we did not examine the term *sick* because it referred specifically to physical rather than mental illness and occurred very infrequently in the interviews. Acadians appear to describe mental illness by using other words — *troubled, depressed, disturbed* and the like — while the Irish refer to the mentally ill person as *sick*.

The terms *sick* and *sickness* are examined together because they have the same etymological root and are very close if not identical in the meaning attributed to them. It should be noted first of all that this concept is applied to two forms of illness: ordinary or physical illness, and the other form of illness suffered by people who are "really sick" — the mentally ill. These people are described by the following words: *mental troubles, mental sickness, sick minds* . These terms constitute both a diagnosis and a label attached to certain people. The elements of seriousness and permanence in the term *really sick* are also noteworthy. The diagnosis is based on an individual's acts; people who are mentally "sick" are distinguished by their behaviour, which can be dangerous:

I've heard that they'll try, because they're sick, they'll pull some stunts off where they could injure or kill themselves, you know, because they're really too mentally ill to know what the heck they're doing or they might just pick something up and throw it at somebody or a knife and kill somebody...

Another participant explained that these people "are just in a trance, you speak to them and you don't get through to them at all."

This perception of the mentally ill as possessed dates back to the Middle Ages. When Father Juan Galiberto Jofre founded Europe's first "hospital dels folls" (hospital for the mad) in Valencia in 1409, he said that these people were possessed. The analogy persists: social exclusion and spiritual reintegration. Only the agents have changed, as Thomas Szasz reminds us: the psychiatrist has been substituted for the priest.

The "sick" person is perceived as someone lacking in ability to understand and in individual and social responsibility. Since the acts such a person is suspected of being capable of are feared, an element of control enters the picture. In this sense, the issue is less what "sick" people actually do than what they are believed capable of doing; the potential danger is as threatening as the reality, if not more. Thus, it is permissible to control them through preventive action. Worse yet, one cannot run the risk of letting them remain free. They have to be confined.

According to the participants, a person suffering from mental sickness appears to have the condition for a long time, even for life. Hence, it is necessary to intervene, and a variety of forms of care are suggested, ranging from understanding to confinement. However, for "really sick" people, given the individual and social danger they represent, the psychiatric institution is the only possible solution. The asylum is thus presented as a place where these people can be hidden, forcibly confined and treated. Faced with sickness, the only possibility is to make sure that sick people will not be seen and to treat them out of view:

It just wasn't the thing to do, to show your mentally retarded or sick kid around. Keep him hidden, keep him away.

On the other hand, the participants seem aware of the kind of treatment that institutions prescribe:

It seems inhuman, you know, and you see movies, uh, lots of movies will glorify anything, heh, but you see a movie on mental health or mental sickness, whatever, in these provincial homes or whatever, and you say, my Jesus, it's not human.

These citations suggest some tendencies in the Irish perception of sickness, notably the social obligation to hide deviants. In addition, behaviour to be repressed is emphasized rather than causes of the sickness. Finally, the association between the word *sick* and the word *ill*, described in the next section, should be noted. In sum, the Irish community establishes a medical diagnosis of "sick" primarily on the basis of acts that are judged to be unacceptable.

"Mentally ill"

Like *sick*, this term is used to describe people suffering from illness, but the element of danger — either to the person who is ill or to others — recurs more regularly in this case. People suffering from mental illness are considered crazy, "out of their minds"; they are described as people who cannot function or think. They must also be kept hidden because of the shame associated with this form of illness. However, as a result of medical progress, the mentally ill person is now considered treatable, so that it is not as shameful a condition as it once was:

When I got to thinking about it, and thinking about the advances they've made in handling, you know, over the years, advances they've made in handling mental illnesses or retarded people, they're treating it as a disease now, it's treated today, it's looked upon as a disease, it's not something to be ashamed of any more really, you know.

One participant pointed out that if everyone suffering from mental illness was confined, half the country would be locked up. He concluded that only people who committed reprehensible acts were confined; for example, someone who hit his mother should be committed to a psychiatric institution.

The Irish do not devote much attention to explaining the reasons for this condition: only two participants addressed this question, citing an accident or a previous illness. The expression *he has mental illness* suggests the congenital nature of the condition.

In the case of both terms that recurred frequently in the interviews *sick* and *mental illness* — the emphasis is placed on the potential threat that these "deviants" represent. Because they are incapable of sober, predictable conduct, they are excluded by being hidden at home or in an institution. The descriptions relating to both terms concentrate more on actions than on causes. In this way, the Irish view is close to the medical model for explaining deviance and differs from the Acadian explanation, which tries to relate the cause of abnormal states to events in normal life.

Having presented the two concepts most often used to designate the mentally ill, we will examine in greater detail the forms that mental illness can take and the ways people suffering from it are described. First, however, we will look at the forms of therapy suggested for mental illness.

6.3.2 Analysis of Terms Designating a Therapeutic Relationship

"Help"

This term was not used frequently in the interviews; it is highlighted because of the system it belongs to and its potential for comparison with other groups. It is used to signify individual or social assistance to a person experiencing emotional problems rather than material or financial aid.

The greatest help I could get for my husband was if he had somebody come in and talk to him, that would talk to him about the things that he wanted to talk about and that he enjoyed.

This concept suggests moral support and an informal, noninstitutional, nonprofessional network of assistance.

"Care"

This term is used in the sense of "take care" of someone and thus means almost the same thing as *help*. *Care* is a positive form of assistance in time of need. The term denotes a degree of warmth and closeness between people. Its significance can perhaps best be seen when it is used in the negative sense: the expression *doesn't care* refers to an indifferent, remote person.

The family and even the psychiatric institution can fill these needs, at least up to a point. One participant even argued that hiding someone could constitute a form of care:

As you got older and became senile in that sense, the family always took care of them, while they hid their skeletons in the closet.

The terms *"treat"* and *"treatment"*

The kind of care designated by the terms *treat* and *treatment* can take on several forms. According to the Irish, treatment can be dispensed in the community, a clinic or, most frequently, a psychiatric institution. The people treated in the institution are those suffering from mental illness. The Irish appear to dissociate the term *help* from the term *treat* :

Criteria for putting them away or helping them, or not helping them but treating them.

For the mentally ill, treatment is prescribed. The term has an especially negative connotation in the expression "they treated them quite rough." Treatment can also last a long time — in one case, forty or forty-five years. In general, it involves a system of care, taking charge of an individual once the ineffectiveness of other methods has been acknowledged. The term assumes passive behaviour by the treated person. There is little involvement on the part of the individual, who undergoes treatment, as in the expressions "he was treated," "they treated her." The concept of obligation reinforces this passivity: "They have to be treated." Distance and expertise, rather than closeness and human warmth, are the characteristics of treatment.

It also implies that a person is kept in an institution against his or her will. Treatment of this sort is given to people who are *sick, a real danger, worn out, insane* or *depressed*. By contrast, an alcoholic can be "treated" in an outpatient clinic, and parents can "treat" children who are retarded or suffer from Down's syndrome.

Treatment suggests the same kind of impersonality as the concept of *mental* (see below). It is a kind of "care" characterized by the subject's lack of participation and dependence on the system and by the lack of attention given to causes. Taking charge and passivity go together; in sum, this form of "treatment" is presented as an imposition of values and constraints to protect society rather than to assist an individual.

6.3.3 Analysis of Terms that Designate Mental Illness

"Retarded" and *"Mentally retarded"*

The meaning of these two terms is the same and they can be analysed together. The characteristics of mental retardation are an inability to understand at the same level as an "ordinary" person, and economic, emotional and social dependency.

In general, participants presented this condition as a congenital one and maintained that they could easily recognize people suffering from it by sight. "I can spot, just observe them." Such people remain retarded for life. The only hope for them consists of some forms of education in special schools or the possibility of keeping busy either in school or in a workshop. This is the form of assistance that can be provided to them and is suggested for them.

Parents are ashamed of mentally retarded children, and as a result always keep them hidden. People do not want to see, hear about or talk about the mentally retarded:

They would keep him in the house or keep him sort of, you know, behind closed doors sort of thing and you'd never hear them ever talk about it in these particular families and they were ashamed, it was something they were ashamed of.

Another participant suggested that since the mentally retarded now fall into the category of people who are "ill" and therefore are now integrated into the medical care system, they are no longer a source of shame. They simply have to be entrusted to the care network, like other people who are "ill." This same argument is currently being used to bring psychiatry into the community and take the mentally ill out of the traditional asylum. Psychiatrists now say that the mentally ill should no longer be isolated in a psychiatric institution: there is no longer any need to hide them or be ashamed of them, but they should be entrusted instead to the people responsible for "community psychiatry."

The mentally retarded can also represent danger: "I'm sure most families, if they have a mentally retarded person that's dangerous, would agree that they just can't have him running around shooting at people, trying to kill people." If they are or become dangerous, they have to be confined.

The term *mentally retarded* is usually applied to an individual, but on rare occasions it is also associated with the word *institution*. The participant who made this association questioned the form of therapy recommended for the mentally retarded:

There are special classes that are set up for people and even the mentally retarded school, you know, the whole thing is so screwed up — it's not, uh, you know, scrap the whole thing.

A retarded person who is able to function and to work without disturbing other people is regarded as making a social contribution and therefore as having some value:

I gather he's retarded, I don't know. He works as a labourer for the city. He's not very sociable but he doesn't bother anybody; he studies karate and that sort of thing. He functions, he works, and he doesn't bother anybody.

Mentally retarded people are thus presented as marginals who can be tolerated so long as they are not dangerous. If they work and accept social norms, they become integrated and are tolerated. If they do not, there is a tendency to exclude them. The apprenticeship and care system directed to them is based on a special model of the school system conceived specifically for them.

The word *"nervous"*

The term *nervous* was used only eight times in the interviews and is presented here primarily in comparison with the Acadian expression *sur les nerfs* (a case of nerves), from which it should be carefully distinguished. It is also important to note the double meaning of *nervous*. Used by itself, the term designates a normal person who is unusually excitable, somewhat irritable, less calm than the average. Such people could be described as "high-strung." Nervousness is a minor form of deviance, an abnormal but accepted condition, less serious than depression. Nervous people are betrayed by their actions: thus, they make mistakes when they drive a car.

Association of the term *nervous* with *breakdown* or depression yields a different scenario: a more serious illness that requires treatment. But even in this case, it appears to be a temporary condition and the patient can be brought back to normal through drugs. In the first case, it is essentially a personality trait that is being referred to, while in the second it is a form of depression.

Acadians used the term *sur les nerfs* to refer to a fairly serious condition that required care and institutionalization. Such people were presented as being dangerous.

The word *"depressed"*

This word describes a condition of dejection for which nothing can apparently be done — except perhaps to administer drugs and commit the person in question to an institution. The solution resorted to is involuntary confinement and treatment in a psychiatric institution. One participant reported a case in which a depressed person remained in the institution for forty or forty-five years. In other, less serious cases, the word *depressed* refers to more temporary forms of deviance, the main requirements for which are understanding on the part of those surrounding the person in question and some sedatives, rather than confinement. In cases where the person is "terribly depressed" or "really depressed," an element of danger and the near-impossibility of returning to normal are mentioned:

Well, let's say if they were violent, unable to handle, and sometimes really very depressed and possibly you couldn't do anything with them.

Depression is a condition with a number of degrees of seriousness, ranging from an almost benign, temporary state to one requiring long-term psychiatric hospitalization. If depressed people become violent and un-controllable, confinement becomes a necessity, both for control and for rehabilitation. Another characteristic of depression is that it is reached after passing through preliminary stages: a person can be disturbed, then nervous, and finally depressed. In this sense, the term is close to *discouraged* and *mental*.

The terms *"wrong"* and *"something wrong"*

These concepts refer both to something bad and to evil in the moral sense. In general, they refer to an individual or a behaviour classified as incorrect or marginal. One participant gave as an example people who kill presidents and popes and said there was "something wrong" with people who act in that way. There are "quite a few that are still out, they haven't gotten in there yet," he suggested.

The participants rendered a moral and social judgement on these people, and a verdict of exclusion followed. Their difference was noted and marginalized. These people could be dangerous, they could become wicked, they could kill. They too are recognized by their behaviour, and the diagnosis of *something wrong* appears to be categorical and definitive:

There's something wrong with those people, there must be something wrong with them.

Something wrong is a rather vague concept indicating an individual's incapacity to act according to the norms of the community. These people are regarded as deviant, but just how deviant depends on the acts they commit and the danger they represent. The condition is generally a congenital one: "there *is* something wrong", "something *is* wrong." For this condition as for others, causes are not mentioned, and possible results are described instead.

The forms of control prescribed for these people are drugs and institutionalization. The institution is suggested primarily when someone threatens the peace or the social order.

The term *"crazy"*

The word *crazy* is used to describe madness in a somewhat rough-and-ready, pedestrian, unrefined way. In the terms of our analysis, it would be a synonym for *mentally disturbed* or *mentally ill*.

I don't think crazy is a proper word any more. I don't know what word we should use there but mostly, I suppose it would be mentally disturbed today, wouldn't it?

In the interviews, three different connotations for *crazy* were found. The first of these is similar to the meaning of *wacky* or *nuts*: it quite simply designates an act or a person that is somewhat out of the ordinary. In a more subtle sense, it means the reverse of mad, as in the expression *crazy like a fox*: the person is not crazy at all, despite appearances. The third meaning is a forbidden one: *crazy* is an impolite word that should not be uttered and is not accepted in society. Hence, substitutes are used: more sophisticated expressions such as *mentally ill* or *mentally disturbed*. Thus, the word has a light meaning, a subtle meaning, and finally, a sociomedical meaning that since the coming of psychiatry has been replaced by more scientific concepts.

One participant noted that very few people are normal and every one of us is a little crazy:

The thing is, as I get older, I find that there are not many normal people, you know, everybody's a little bit crazy in some way or another. It's a very grey area.

Whether or not a person categorized as *crazy* can be tolerated depends on the person's actions: "As long as he's acting normally.... He's very responsible at his job and he does his work." Here too, note how the person attains legitimacy through work, and how a greater degree of tolerance is reserved for those who contribute to the market economy.

The participants made no mention of the causes of this condition in the interviews. In essence, it is a category with rather fuzzy boundaries. It is contrasted to *normal*, which is itself a somewhat relative diagnosis. No danger is mentioned in connection with these people, and a positive value is placed on their participation in work.

The term *"insane"*

This term designates a person who is legally mad: people who have committed illegal acts may plead insanity — that is, innocence by virtue of a psychiatric disorder — at their trials. Three of the five participants who used this term mentioned John Hinckley, who had tried to assassinate President Reagan a few months before the interviews, in this connection. People who are insane have no moral feeling, cannot reason ("out of their minds"), and are not responsible for their actions:

I suppose he can't help it so you could call him insane.

People who are insane are considered dangerous, so that in their case there is no alternative to the psychiatric institution and the range of treatments associated with it. As a general rule, they should not be released unless they show that they can take complete responsibility for their actions and are in that sense cured.

The concept is used in a legal context when the notion of individual responsibility arises following an offence. The loss of reason is the primary characteristic of the concept and explains why the person commits illegal acts. It should be noted, however, that some people abuse the recourse to an insanity defence to avoid imprisonment: the accused or their lawyers sometimes choose the psychiatric rather than the judicial route.

Since "insane" people are not responsible for their actions, the community wants to make sure that they will not repeat those actions and expects that they will receive effective treatment in the psychiatric institution:

Until such a time that he can be released to society or not released if he cannot be, if he cannot get any better, you know, if he can be cured we'll say or treated with whatever they treat them with at institutions.

The word *"bad"*

Here too, there is no mention of the cause of the condition, and participants concentrated more on the question of treatment, concluding that confinement is the only acceptable therapy. Behaviour characterized as *bad* is very serious and justifies this form of intervention. Such people must be locked up because they contravene society's limits of tolerance. If society cannot control them, the institution will take it upon itself to do so.

Some of them are maybe so bad, we'll say, I don't know, bad... but are so, in such a state that the only place they can be treated and helped and looked after and fed, probably, clothed, and whatever, are in these institutions.

Nor should any attempt be made to make excuses for them:

Well, what's ever become of that word, they're just plain "bad"? Ha! They find excuses for everybody nowadays.

On the other hand, when the individual learns to conform again it can be taken as a distinct sign of improvement:

As she got older, she got a little house of her own and she wasn't too bad. She wasn't bad; she'd do anything Mother would tell her to do.

The condition exists in a number of degrees of seriousness: "not too bad," "pretty bad," "from bad to worse," "real bad." These terms suggest the progressive nature of the pathology without indicating its causes, which were not explained by any of the participants. The method of choice for controlling these people is still the psychiatric institution, which appears to be the only system that can guarantee that society will be protected. The influence that these people can have should also be noted. If they are not controlled, there is a risk that others will follow them:

They call the local doctors in if somebody goes bad and he wheels away people's spirits that you've read about in books.

The word *"mental"*

The Irish use this word to designate the category of people suffering from the most serious forms of mental illness. The word recurred very frequently in the interviews and was associated with a variety of other terms, as in "mental case", "mental person", "mental problem", "mental institution" ,"mental attitude."

When the term is used, it often involves a judgement or a diagnosis made as a consequence of a way of being or thinking regarded as deviant. The individual is referred to as a "case," just as in the medical world. In the interviews with the Irish, the expression "mental case" recurred twelve times. The word refers to individuals impersonally, like numbers, and places them in pigeonholes:

They traced it way back from where some of her relatives had mental cases.

Generally speaking, "mental" people are neither wicked nor guilty; rather, they cannot control themselves and act incomprehensibly, unacceptably or unusually. Whereas "bad" people were blamed, "mental" ones are not. This does not mean, however, that they are accepted in their environment. On the contrary, they must be sent away, hidden, confined. Living in a traditional society, the Irish in rural areas find it easier to accept the idea of hiding them at home or in a special care home. In industrialized areas, on the other hand, the institution is the location of choice for them. In both cases, the idea is to avoid seeing or hearing "mental" people. They are not blamed for their condition, but the shame they give rise to is felt, and they must be hidden.

In the categories of *mentally ill*, *wrong*, *crazy* and *insane*, it was often feared that the individuals in question would commit dangerous acts. They were locked up to prevent a potential danger from actually happening. Possible actions are mentioned less frequently for this category. "Mental" people disturb others by their condition, and it is necessary to get rid of them:

Well I know people that were put away and they're still away but I mean they were mental, you know.

One participant mentioned that any social judgement of them is subjective:

So you see lots of mental cases there, or apparent mental cases to our way of thinking.

Another participant even referred to them as intelligent:

Of course, mental people are intelligent no doubt too in their own way.

And "mental" was even associated with genius:

Well, I think the difference between a genius and a mental person is a very narrow line.

"Mental" and *"danger"*

The picture of "mental" people presented by the Irish does not appear to be based on either acts or causes, but rather on the danger that a certain category of individuals might represent if they are left free to act as they like. In order to prevent incidents with disagreeable consequences, people who behave in an alien and unacceptable way are excluded. The individuals in question are not blamed; rather, the Irish are bothered by the way they act and the danger they represent. Society cannot allow itself to let a mental person remain free:

They can't be allowed to hurt other people.

The irrationality they represent must be reduced to silence. This idea brings us back to the writing of Michel Foucault: "From having been a consequence, the disappearance of freedom becomes the foundation, the inner reason, the essence of madness. And the restrictions that must be imposed on the material freedom of the insane are prescribed by this essence."[4]

There are two major ways in which the Irish recognize "mental" cases: they have little or no cognitive ability and little or no ability to adapt to existing norms. A person who goes for a walk in the nude, for example, is defying a norm.

Two forms of treatment for this deviance recurred regularly in the interviews: the institution, which serves the purpose of control, and drugs, which are directed towards essentially the same end. According to one participant:

These days they give them pills to keep them kind of quiet. As long as they take their medication, they're all right.

The word *mental* was used along with a reference to the institution nine times, in the following forms: *mental hospital, mental place, mental health, mental institution.* The previous comments in this regard (see section 6.2.2) apply here as well. The term *treatment* recurred regularly in association with the "mental institution." In addition, one participant described the institution as a refuge when family and social stress become untenable.

6.3.4 Conclusion

On the basis of the interviews, the conception of assistance held by the Irish oscillates between two poles. First, there is a family and social network characterized by the terms *help* and *care* in which assistance is personal and local and responds to the needs of individuals. However, when this form of assistance is not enough and it is necessary to introduce an element of individual control to prevent potentially dangerous situations, the term *treatment* comes into play, implying protection for society at least as much as the hope that the individual will be cured.

The system of deviance in the Irish community is characterized by shame and refusal to allow an abnormal person to appear in public. In rural areas, "mental," "retarded" or "crazy" people would be hidden at home or sometimes in an institution. In industrial settings, there is a greater tendency to use the institution as a means of hiding such people.

Unlike the Acadians, the Irish do not show much interest in the causes of deviance. The Irish appear to have a more medicalized approach to deviance: they diagnose and prescribe treatment to eliminate the symptom. Few participants looked back at the social factors that might cause deviance. As the Irish see it, the subject must clearly conform and adhere to social norms. Social control is exercised through inner-directedness, to use David Riesman's term.

The Irish appear to be afraid not of the danger as such that these people represent but of the threat of danger. Thus, the Irish do not say very much about what people suffering from mental illness actually do; instead, they talk about how they will eventually lose their faculties. In this case, the community takes responsibility for individual control by finding ways of predicting and preventing embarrassing or dangerous situations. The concept of shame that arose several times at the family level appears to operate here as well: people are ashamed not only of deviants but also of those who could become deviants.

Having examined each of the words contained in the analysis, we can now set up a schema describing the representation of mental illness in the Irish community (figure 13). The inner circle (A) indicates that the essence of the representation of mental illness centres on the word *mental*. Circle B shows the different concepts associated with *mental* in the interviews, along with the frequency of these associations. The largest circle (C) shows indirect relationships and more distant associations among concepts. Words in this circle indicate forms of deviance that are less serious and less intimately related to *mental*. Finally, the square indicates the system of care that is generally prescribed for these pathologies. As the abnormality becomes more serious, it becomes more closely related to the mind (*mens, mental*) and institutional treatment becomes more likely to be seen as the only solution. On the other hand, farther away from the centre a different set of needs becomes involved, moving gradually

Figure 13
Summary of How the Irish
Perceive Mental Illness

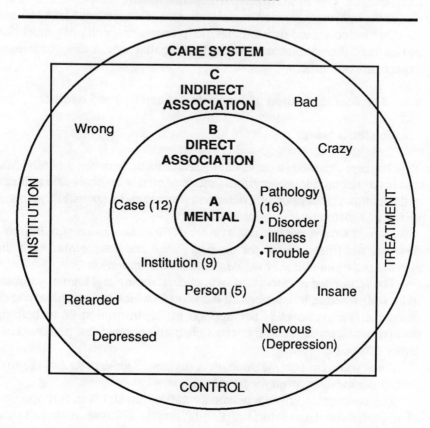

towards an approach based on care and help, as these terms are conceived by the Irish community.

6.4 RESULTS OF INTERVIEWS WITH THE LOYALISTS

It was quite difficult to recruit candidates of Loyalist origin in the city of Moncton because the group has no formal organization in the region and does not live in a well-defined area. It was necessary to proceed through local history teachers and writers. Five candidates agreed to be interviewed.

Both in Moncton and in Salisbury, where another five people were interviewed, a number of Loyalist participants were clearly very suspicious. One participant in Salisbury agreed to an interview but refused to let it be taped. One of the urban participants, having been informed of the aim of the interview, wanted to make sure that the tape would not be used for other purposes and insisted that the interviewer specify his intentions in this regard on the tape itself; only after that would this participant express his opinions.

6.4.1 The Medicalization of Deviants as Seen by the Loyalists

The term *"care"*

This concept describes a dependency relationship between an individual and his or her immediate environment. It primarily involves care at home and contains a presupposition of human warmth and responsibility; in this sense, it is differentiated from *treatment* :

I would say people that can't be cared for at home, their family don't have the facilities to care for them at home and people that need the specialized treatment they would get in an institution.

The term *care* is associated with understanding and human warmth; in its widest sense, it describes all the ways in which an individual can be cared for. The concept is not applied to the institution or to helping professionals; on the contrary, a participant mentioned that professionals rarely offer care:

Once you went into the door of an asylum ... unless you met the rare type of doctor who cared for people ...

The concept describes a personal relationship and is in fact opposed to a professional or institutional relationship because it describes a community-based rather than institutional form of assistance in case of need.

The word *"help"*

This word is used to describe a number of levels of assistance in case of need: in its traditional meaning, it refers to support, comfort and love as they are found in a family:

They had given me all the support and all the love and all the help, but something else had happened.

This term also refers to the assistance people can receive from professionals, such as counselling. It is also said that drugs "help" people to control their mental illness and put them back into a position to function normally. Finally, a psychiatrist can offer "help," and the psychiatric institution can sometimes "help" an individual. Although the concept is applied to a number of forms of assistance, it appears to be primarily associated with professional intervention.

But the help was ignorant and biased and the poor souls got pushed around and knocked around because the government didn't spend enough money to have educated help.

Participants believe that the institution "helps" people, or at least that there is no reason to believe the reverse. A person who comes out of the institution has been "helped." Drugs also constitute a form of help. However, it is worth noting that a pharmacist who was part of the sample emphasized the repressive value of the pharmaceutical products he sells: "Well it keeps them quiet I sure think, but it doesn't help."

People in rural regions tend to associate help with its traditional aspect, which includes talking, loving, being there. In urban areas, the same term is more likely to imply an external, professional network. It is in urban areas that such concepts as *educated help* and *paid help* are found. Thus, the concept of help encompasses a number of services, a number of forms and conceptions of assistance. At one extreme is the traditional, family notion of help, with its community network. At the other extreme are professional mental health services, medicalization and confinement in a psychiatric institution.

The words *"treat"* and *"treatment"*

These words are sometimes associated with *help* and *care*, but are distinguished by the form of assistance they involve: institutional rather than personal and family responsibility. Thus, "but in the home, they weren't treating...her." A number of participants emphasized the fact that dangerous people need "treatment":

Almost for their protection and also for the protection of others that they should be — but given treatment, not just locked away and left.

The psychiatrist is also an agent of treatment:

I'd like to see more psychiatrists be hired by the government so that they can treat these people better when they're in the institution and it's possible that they could have extramural treatment for these too.

The dissociation between *treatment* and *care* should be noted here. People are treated inside the institution; when they get out, they are cared for. Sometimes, the family or community network takes on the role of an agent of treatment, and the expressions *treat them all right* and *treated with sympathy* can be interpreted in this way. *Treatment* in this sense is close to the concepts of *help* and *care* studied previously. In general, however, the term tends to describe an external, dictated approach. People have no choice but to "get treatment" when they suffer from certain mental illnesses:

If they've got a mental illness I don't think that they can make the choice not to be treated or not to be put in a place where they can't harm themselves or somebody else.

The expression *go for treatment* also indicates the compulsory, passive nature of the process of taking responsibility for the individual. In sum, when social and community agencies attach a diagnosis to an individual, they also prescribe an appropriate method of treatment at the same time. When all other approaches have failed, there is no form of treatment left except the psychiatric institution. In this sense, the institution is not even necessarily a place where people are treated. Thus, "They're just put away and when they come out they just do the same thing because they never were treated..." Similarly, a person must go to the psychiatric institution "when it's hopeless, when there's no treatment, when you're too late for treatment or treatment won't help you any."

Some participants believe that as the mentally ill have become medicalized, their "treatment" has improved. Before, committing the mentally ill to a psychiatric institution was the only option when the situation was serious; now, at least there is a choice between drugs and confinement. The participants seem more favourably disposed towards the first solution:

Yes, they were put there and you felt that ... you know, there was no help for them and I guess if truth were known there wasn't a great deal of help for them. But I think there is now what with a greater knowledge, better medications and better treatments.

Treatment was associated a number of times with *shock*, in reference to electroconvulsive therapy. Participants' comments on this form of therapy were unfavourable; they pictured it as dictated, barbaric and ineffective:

There was a lady who lived in the same house with us who had a nervous breakdown and she was in there and they gave her shock treatments and I remember when she came home, she looked like a zombie, you know —just didn't seem to really be aware of too much, you know.

The concept of treatment thus encompasses a number of forms of assistance and points to a number of possibilities for intervention. These possibilities include traditional methods and run the gamut from natural foods and vitamins through involving a doctor and committing the patient to an institution all the way to electroconvulsive therapy. Most participants, however, associated *treatment* with the institution. In such cases, the term becomes a synonym for a form of protective custody rather than personal intervention aimed at helping the individual. When there is danger to society, the institution serves to protect both the individual and those around her or him, and this protection is also referred to as *treatment*.

If it's an organic cause that cannot be treated at home and, you know, if they can't be handled, if there's a possibility of them becoming violent and harming people, then they definitely have to be put somewhere where they're going to be safe.

It is noteworthy here that the reference is to potential rather than real danger. A person who is capable of violent acts must be treated and confined — treated by being confined.

The three terms *care*, *help* and *treatment* constitute a frame of reference for dealing with abnormality in Loyalist society. The more threatening the individual, the more likely it is that coercive forms of intervention will be resorted to. When the situation cannot be stabilized in any other way, candidates are committed to the institution, for their own protection or for the protection of others.

We will now look at the terms that refer to deviance as used by Loyalist participants in describing various manifestations of mental illness.

6.4.2 Semantic Analysis of Terms Designating Mental Illness

The word *"trouble"*

The term *trouble* occurred only four times, but it is worth analysing briefly, primarily for purposes of comparison with the other groups. In general it refers to an individual whose behaviour does not conform to the established norm. The forms of behaviour involved, however, appear rather benign when compared with, say, *trouble* as viewed by the Acadians. In the Loyalists' perception, such people can cause their parents "quite a lot of trouble," can be "expelled" from school, and in general, need "a psychologist" or some other form of "counselling."

An adolescent causes some trouble for his parents during a critical period, or a slightly disturbed child troubles his parents' life and his school environment.

I have a very close friend, she's been having trouble with her little boy, she herself has been going to a psychologist to get help for him.

Trouble is a relatively mild form of deviance characterized by the failure of the individual's behaviour to conform to the social rules of daily life. It does not have the same meaning for the Loyalists as for the Acadians; it is disturbing, but in a temporary and relatively superficial way.

The terms *"nerves"* and *"nervous"*

These terms have two different meanings. First, they refer to people with a case of *nerves* or a *nervous condition.* These people are born that way and are unable to control their own actions. They need tranquilizers — drugs that will help regulate their behaviour.

If such a condition gets worse, it is referred to as a *mental breakdown* or *nervous breakdown.* This can happen for a variety of reasons: a hormonal imbalance, the accidental death of a loved one, or "working too hard." In other words, it is a situational form of deviance. The Loyalists see electroconvulsive therapy as the treatment of choice for problems of this sort. If the situation really becomes serious, it is necessary to resort to confinement in a psychiatric institution — although participants were aware of the limitations of this solution:

I think when you know someone ... who has a nervous breakdown or something like that, you feel, well, they are wasting their lives in these mental institutes.

As Michel Foucault noted, techniques last longer than the reasons for them. One participant pointed out some difficulties that people who come out of such an institution have to face:

You could have a nervous breakdown and get over it but if you were bad enough to have been sent to these places, why you'd soon be back again for the way people looked at you and whispered about you and so on.

People described as *nervous* or having a case of *nerves* are born that way and have to live with their handicap while taking drugs to keep themselves under control. A person who has a *nervous breakdown*, on the other hand, is regarded as suffering from a more serious but temporary condition.

The word *"sick"*

In contrast to the word *ill*, the term *sick* specifically designates someone whose disease is located in the mind. People used to be described as *crazy* and identified as such by their actions; thus, "she acts crazy." Now, there is a greater tendency to use the word *sick*, but it is the individual who is sick and not his or her actions. One participant explained the difference between these two conceptions in the following terms: "Crazy to me is a word that's...about a person that acts silly rather than a person that is sick." The "sick" person is considered dangerous and is capable of violence:

I think that ... people who commit crimes like murder and that sort of thing is called temporary insanity but if it happens once it can happen again and I feel those people are sick, that they are definitely sick, that there is something wrong with a person that does that.

In all the interviews, only one participant mentioned a cause for a person's becoming sick: working too hard. On the basis of the forms of intervention recommended for this condition, it is considered a very serious one: participants believe that sick people need "care" and "treatment." Madness is now in the domain of illness; according to the current medical approach, the individual must be cared for and treated. People used to concentrate on actions without necessarily condemning the person who committed them; now, there is a greater tendency to talk about the person who is sick.

The term *"stupid"*

This is a term that people nowadays hesitate to use, preferring to substitute more medically-oriented expressions:

Stupid is a word that was used more when I was small — growing up. Everybody was stupid. I mean, that was very popular. I don't hear that word now—being stupid. Now we're getting more cultivated and civilized.

There is a noteworthy expression associated with this term. A stupid person is one who, without realizing it, "is not dealing with a full deck of cards." It is not without irony that one participant mentioned that people who are responsible for taking care of patients in psychiatric institutions are themselves "stupid":

Send someone you love to a place like that knowing you can't handle them but you also know some stupid, ignorant person is going to be responsible for them.

Like the term *crazy*, *stupid* is less a part of the spoken language than it used to be, having been replaced by other terms that are both more medically-oriented and more subtle:

Crazy and stupid, I mean, that was our vocabulary. But now, like I said, we're getting civilized through television and we're getting more educated so now they're not crazy, they're mentally ill, you see. And, of course, sometimes if we're really smart we'll really put other labels on them like they're psychotic or they're hypochondriac or they're schizophrenic or they're paranoid.

The expression *"something wrong"*

This term is a modifier used to condemn an action or a way of being or acting. In essence, it is the opposite of *normal*, but both of these terms are quite vague. People with whom there is "something wrong" can be recognized as such by their actions: people who are compulsive, criminals, people who "do foolish things." Such people cannot reason or use their heads like the rest of us:

It would be somebody that can't behave rationally. If there's something wrong with his or her mind so that they can't reason rationally, they do foolish things, make their hands go in foolish ways, and they get rather rough physically with some people with whom they come in contact.

Their minds don't seem to work well. Participants concentrated on obvious manifestations, external signs, forms of behaviour that indicate an internal abnormality. They described such people as "not normal" and as "mentally ill." Here again it is the person, and not only his or her behaviour, that comes under attack. The highly subjective nature of this judgement is worth noting. The case of an adolescent who read too much and was given electroshock treatments because her behaviour bothered her mother is a good example:

Her mother felt that she was very strange because she would sit and read and her mother sent her to a psychologist when she was a teenager. That I think had a very bad effect on her, she had shock treatment ... She was normal, she liked to sit and read and enjoy being by herself but her mother had been a very outgoing person, couldn't understand this.

The institution is the only form of therapy recommended for this category.

The word *"bad"*

This term is used both for a physical ailment ("a bad back") and for a form of behaviour categorized as immoral or wicked. In the latter case, what is involved is a form of deviance caused by a nervous condition. Nerves can be "bad"; if the condition becomes serious, however, the only realistic solution is to commit the person who has become "bad" because of bad nerves. Such a person can be dangerous; one participant reported the example of a man who killed his wife and had to be committed. In this case, the sudden, unpredictable element in the man's behaviour is worth noting: "All of a sudden, he went bad."

The experience of people who have to spend time in an institution is characterized as "bad" in the sense that when they get out again, they are banished from society: they are ostracized. It is implied here that it is not only these individuals who are bad but also the people around them who pass judgement on the victims on the basis of their having spent time in a psychiatric institution.

This term describes a nervous condition that can be manifested in threatening acts by the individual, who then becomes categorized as "bad." Such people were once hidden away at home: "I think fifty years ago they did hide it." Now, they are confined in an institution. Even though the place of confinement has changed, the approach remains the same. Once a family responsibility, estrangement of the individual to preserve the social order has now become the responsibility of the state.

The word *"crazy"*

Although participants maintained that this word is hardly ever used any more, it occurred thirty-one times in the nine interviews with the Loyalists. It is used, first of all, in a light sense to refer to the "crazy" part of us that we all have to let out to maintain our equilibrium: "We have a silly statement in our house and we'll say that we're crazy, it keeps us from going insane."

The term is also used in a much more serious sense to refer to someone who is irrational and commits unreasonable actions. The individual is described through these actions: such a person rapes, performs all sorts of deviant sexual acts, kills. It was a crazy person, for example, who tried to kill President Reagan. Participants used the term to describe someone regarded as seriously perturbed. One maintained that it is the worst of all conditions: "Yes, I don't know of anything worse in that line that I can think of that would be extremely crazy."

The only treatment mentioned for this condition was the straitjacket:

To me the word crazy means someone who is so mentally deranged that he has to be put in a straitjacket.

At one time, madness was not associated with illness; instead, it was regarded as a "horrible affliction," a kind of social curse something like leprosy. Now, medicine has tamed madness by explaining it scientifically, so madness falls into its area of competence. One participant maintained that as a result of our education we can now think about this subject in a more professional way. Thus, we now understand madness better and we can treat it sympathetically instead of being afraid of it. At no time were any causes mentioned for this form of deviance. Participants concentrated more on describing the kinds of action and speech that characterize people regarded as crazy.

La Fontaine said of the plague that not everyone died of it but everyone was affected by it. The same comment could apply to madness. We all have a bit of latent madness in us that threatens us and can be detected through certain signs:

You can take a person who's been absolutely normal all their life and then something will happen, you know ...They go crazy or they just go to pieces and maybe they're admitted to a hospital or something like this. Really, you know, it's not something they're born with, it's just something that happens. It could happen to either one of us.

Madness is threatening; it might show. It must be contained; scandal must be avoided; it can't be allowed to become contagious. As Michel Foucault has written:

Homo medicus was ... called into the world of confinement ... to protect others from the vague danger that exuded through the walls of confinement ... If a doctor was summoned, if he was asked to observe, it was because people were afraid ...The ideal was an asylum which ... would have all the powers of example and none of the risks of contagion.[5]

The term *"insane"*

This term refers to much the same set of characteristics as it does among the Irish. Thus, it designates a person who has committed an illegal act, such as a murder. Instead of being sent to prison, the insane person is committed. The sentence is an indefinite one and the individual's release depends on the recommendation of the psychiatric and institutional authorities.

One participant suggested that the insane should be dealt with by giving them "care," but a number of others considered them dangerous and saw a lengthy period of confinement as the only possible solution. It is noteworthy that the term *insane* was twice used to describe the institution: "we called it the insane asylum."

Individuals suffering from insanity in the legal sense are regarded as dangerous and often as criminals. They are identified by their actions — visible signs of a temporary or permanent loss of reason.

The word *"depression"*

This term occurred eleven times in the nine interviews and was used exclusively by participants from industrialized areas. It is apparently not part of the vocabulary of rural people.

Depression is described as a state brought on by an organic condition. In this sense the cure for it could consist of a better diet, enough rest, and the like. Here too, however, the participants tended to concentrate on describing what they considered dangerous actions that depressed people could carry out: they could let themselves die of hunger or kill themselves and were in general difficult to control. The solutions in which they put their trust were drugs, confinement and electroconvulsive therapy — although they were aware that the effectiveness of this last method was only relative:

I know of people, they gave them shocks — this woman for twenty years that I knew and she came out and got well several times.

In other cases, the impossibility of curing depressed people was acknowledged:

There was another person they couldn't do anything with. She had depressions. She tried to kill herself one time and it was caused by — she got depressions.

In using the term *depression*, participants were referring to a serious condition that can manifest itself in dangerous ways and can be controlled only with appropriate therapy, which often must be imposed on the patient.

The word *"mental"*

This term occurred very frequently in the interviews, more frequently than all other terms used to designate madness — 155 times in the nine interviews. For purposes of analysis, its use was divided into five separate categories.

• *The term* mental *used by itself:*

Used in this way, *mental* describes a person with a permanent, congenital handicap: "people who are born with a handicap and are mental." Such people are described as irresponsible and immature. However, one participant noted that the line separating the sane person from the "mental" one was not very clear:

It is sickness, that's for sure, it's nothing else, 'cause a lot of cases it's a nervous condition that causes it. Just as we say there's a thin line between being sane and mental. Only just a snap and that's it.

As for a solution, two participants mentioned that "mental" people had to be hidden if no institution was available:

They hid those mental — those people of low — I'm talking about an imbecile. They kept them home and kept them hidden in an attic or something and never let them out. There was no institution.

• *The mental person:*

The word *mental* was associated with a person on a number of occasions (*mentally ill person, mental patient*). Such people cannot control themselves and are difficult to take care of. They are potential criminals and cannot be trusted. Here we see the idea of prevention that suggests mistrust towards people who may act abnormally. In this sense, it is necessary to cure through prevention. Keeping someone under supervision becomes a form of intervention based on prevention or perhaps mistrust.

• *The "mentally retarded" person:*

Like the other groups, the Loyalists frequently associate this term with children, although they say that mentally retarded people are incapable of learning anything:

She went to school for fifteen years and in those fifteen years she learned nothing. She was labelled mentally retarded.

These people can be recognized by their appearance: a local expression to describe them is that they are "a few bricks shy of a load." The Loyalists feel pity towards people suffering from mental retardation, as they live a sad life. The system of *help* mentioned previously is considered an appropriate solution. It is also believed that these people should be kept at home even if their condition is permanent and incurable.

• *The institution associated with the term* mental:

Four expressions are grouped under this heading: *mental institution, mental institute, mental health* and *mental hospital*. My previous comments about the juxtaposition of the words *mental* and *institution* (see section 6.2.2) apply here as well. The "mental institution" is a place where subjects whose behaviour deviates from the norm are sent: for example, a person who sleeps under the bed rather than in the bed.

In the nineteenth century, the director of a psychiatric institution said that "no insane man recovers at home." This kind of thinking still appears to be prevalent, if one participant's view is any indication:

The family has a tendency to keep people that they shouldn't. ... They should put them in a mental institution.

On the other hand, a number of participants were aware of the institutional malaise that hangs over people who are committed: "If they didn't die in the first week they lived a good long while." Psychiatric institutions were also described as a "pure waste of time." Moreover, participants were aware that people could be admitted to them for rather dubious reasons:

Do you remember there was a man in a mental hospital for years and years and years? And the only reason he was there was that he was speaking a language that nobody understood and they thought the man was seriously deranged.

The way in which the Loyalists describe the psychiatric institution indicates that they recognize its limits and even its harmful effects. Thus, participants were quite critical of such institutions. It is also worth noting that the terms *care* and *help* were never associated with *institution*. On the other hand, the concepts of temporary or permanent observation and electroconvulsive therapy were associated with it, confirming our previous description of the role of the institution.

• *"Mental" pathology:*

Terms indicating a pathology associated with the word *mental* — such as *mental problem, mentally deranged, mentally ill, mentally handicapped, mental disability*, to name only the more significant ones — have been grouped under this heading.

These are conditions which do not allow individuals to live independently or take responsibility for themselves because of their state of mind. In this sense, these individuals are deviant and sick. An institutional system must therefore be set up to take care of them, especially when they are considered dangerous. Here too, the danger is potential rather than real. A person who cannot function autonomously but does not constitute a serious danger should be watched rather than confined:

Now, not all mentally ill people, I don't feel, have to be put in an institution. If they can function without harming themselves or anybody else and if somebody is willing to oversee them—you know, make sure that they're eating properly and getting along.

Some participants acknowledged that the community defines mental pathology and imposes confinement in a psychiatric institution somewhat arbitrarily.

You know, she is a very smart lady although she is definitely mentally ill because her family definitely feels this and I think that the doctor in the end felt that the family is trying to have her put away.

Thus, the community, the family and professionals all contribute towards defining marginality and excluding people. No more detail is given, however, about the specific responsibility of each of these. Possible solutions to mental pathology range from the use of vitamins through drugs and clinical help to the institution. Most participants favoured this last solution:

There are people that if badly mentally ill, I think they're more at home in an institution that is set for them maybe because there's people that they can identify with more.

A number of causes for mental pathology were suggested: inbreeding, senility, drug abuse, a nervous temperament, an accident. In the ninety-two times that mental pathology was mentioned, there were only six attempts to identify a cause. This indicates that little importance is attached to causes. Participants concentrated more on describing conditions, solutions and people's reactions.

6.4.3 Conclusion

The preceding are the salient points in Loyalist participants' perception of mental illness. The terms *care, help* and *treatment* recur, as they do among the Irish. However, the Loyalists resort to treatment more quickly and more categorically than the Irish do. Each of the three terms is applied to a particular condition and context. As the situation becomes more difficult and the individual becomes more uncontrollable (at least potentially), there is a greater tendency to look towards confinement in the institution as a solution.

From the terms the Loyalists use most frequently to categorize and describe mental illness, a system of perception of mental illness can be identified for the group. This system centres on the term *mental*. The closer we get to this term, the more the individual in question is considered dangerous. The method of treatment then becomes the institution, for the protection both of the individual and of society.

The realization that all the terms used to describe madness revolve around a social, legal or medical judgement of an individual pathology makes it easier to understand the widespread use of involuntary institutionalization in New Brunswick. In this way, committing individuals who are considered either dangerous or sick can be justified. And if those who are potentially crazy or potentially dangerous are thrown in as well, society runs the risk of becoming very suspicious and intolerant of deviance and deviants. The Loyalists present them with the following choice: dictated social control, or else either bringing their marginality into line or rejecting it.

Participants were aware of the limitations and reputation of the psychiatric institution. The contradiction between the institution's usefulness to society as a means of protection and the relative nature of its value as a means of helping victims is a recurring theme in the analysis. In talking about mental illness, people appear to acknowledge the impossibility of helping individual victims of confinement while at the same time protecting the society that rejects them. Figure 14 is an attempt to show, in graphic form, the characteristics of the various aspects of deviance as they appear in Loyalists' speech. In the "causes" column, the lack of importance accorded to causes by Loyalist participants as compared with, say, the Acadians (see figure 12, p. 118) is noteworthy. It is also worth noting that the Loyalists regard the system of care and help described at the beginning of this chapter as having little applicability to the various categories of deviants. There is little sign of the concepts of help and care to assist marginals, who are entrusted to the institution and professional staff instead. Thus, there is constant reference to the need for treatment and institutionalization. To a greater extent than among the Acadians and Irish, deviance is taken in hand by medical and institutional powers. Since most categories of deviants are considered dangerous, institutionalization becomes necessary more frequently than it does with the other two groups.

Figure 14
Features, Causes and Needs of Various
Mental Illnesses as Seen by the Loyalists

Condition	Features	Causes	Needs
Trouble	• Temporary • Related to problems in everyday life	—	• Attention • Help
Nervous Condition	• Congenital	• Heredity	• Drugs
Nervous breakdown	• Temporary	• Overwork • Accident • Death of loved one	• Electroshock treatment • Institution
Sick	• Dangerous • Capable of violence	• Overwork	• Care • Treatment (in institution)
Stupid	• Popular term referring to madness	—	—
Something wrong	• Dangerous	—	—
Bad	• Unpredictable • Very dangerous	• Bad nerves	• Isolation at home or in institution
Crazy	• Irrational acts • Dangerous illness • Contagious	—	• Straitjacket
Depression	• Danger to self and others	• Organic	• Drugs • Confinement • Electroshock treatment
Insane	• Illegal acts • Very dangerous	—	• Institution for life
Mentally retarded	• Can't learn • Congenital	—	• School • Care
Mental (in other contexts)	• Dangerous	• Senility • Drugs • Accident, etc.	• Institution • Observation

6.5 COMPARISON OF PARTICIPANTS ACCORDING TO PLACE OF RESIDENCE

I will briefly analyse the interviews by grouping them under the headings "rural" and "industrialized."

6.5.1 The Concept of "Work"

My first working hypothesis suggested the need to explore the relationship between mental illness and lack of productivity or inability to work. What little evidence could be gathered on this question is presented here. In the interviews with people living in Moncton, there were sixteen instances where participants referred to the concept of work. Here are a few examples.   '

I gather he's retarded ... He works as a labourer for the city ... He studies karate and that sort of thing. He functions, he works.

He was fired from his job because he was disturbing the others, because he was fooling around.

In the interviews with participants living in rural areas, there were six references to work:

Since she can't live an ordinary life and work, she is mentally ill.

The child could have made a living, he could have worked, but they passed him off as crazy.

Given the relatively small number of references to this theme, no firm conclusions can be drawn. It is nevertheless worth noting that participants living in an industrialized area referred to work almost three times as often as those living in rural areas, reflecting a greater concern with this topic by the industrialized population. Work appears to be one of the litmus tests, one of the criteria people — especially in industrialized areas — use to decide whether to be concerned with particular individuals or whether to exclude them by committing them to psychiatric institutions.

6.5.2 The Term "Danger"

As already noted, this term occurs very frequently in association with mental illness and institutionalization. In some cases, danger was mentioned explicitly: killing, hitting someone with a dangerous instrument, danger to the individual, danger to others, and so forth.

You can't let them go free, because they could kill someone.

The ones who are shooting presidents and popes and things...

If he's potentially violent, you have to lock him up.

A citation was regarded as reflecting a concern with danger only if the element of danger was mentioned explicitly. The frequency with which terms indicating danger occurred is shown in table 16.

Table 16
Frequency of Use of Terms Involving Danger by Ethnic Group and Place of Residence

Ethnic Group	Rural	Industrialized
Loyalists	13	19
Irish	9	7
Acadians	11	6
Total	**33**	**32**

References to the stereotype of the dangerous mentally ill person were considerably more frequent among the Loyalists than among the other two groups. For the Loyalists, the concern with danger is more prevalent among people living in an industrialized area, while the reverse is true for the other two groups. Overall, the sixty-five references to the danger posed by the mentally ill indicate a significant concern with this topic on the part of the participants. Everything indicates that this factor plays a large role in the decision to hospitalize a person involuntarily, and the observations made in analysing the three groups' views of mental health are confirmed.

NOTES

1. Laurence Bardin, *L'Analyse de contenu* (Paris: Presses Universitaires de France, 1977), p. 39.
2. Ibid., p. 4.
3. See Virginia Satir, *Conjoint Family Therapy: A Guide to Theory and Technique* (Palo Alto, Calif.: Science and Behavior Books, 1964).
4. Michel Foucault, *Histoire de la folie à l'âge classique* (Paris: Gallimard, 1972), p. 459.
5. Michel Foucault, *Madness and Civilization* (London: Tavistock Publications, 1965), pp. 205-7.

7
Comparative Analysis of the Interviews

The remarks that follow are aimed at clarifying the results of the content analysis. Through the indicators examined in this chapter, we will be able to obtain an overview of the way the three groups under study perceive mental illness.

The method we chose was designed to use a series of expressions of opinion to interpret the phenomenon of exclusion on grounds of madness of individuals and social categories rejected by the group. We must now identify the major trends that show up in the interviews with a view towards perceiving some common denominators that relate directly or indirectly to our working hypotheses and the general orientation of our research. The three ethnic groups interviewed present different perspectives on madness and different conceptions of what is unacceptable and what is marginal. Some common features, however, stand out in the analysis.

7.1 POINTS OF CONVERGENCE

7.1.1 The Concept of Danger

Each group has a threshold of tolerance towards deviance — psychiatric or other — that stands out clearly in the texts. While these levels of tolerance vary, the element of danger often tips the balance in favour of the protection of society at the expense of the person who is categorized as sick. Everyone seems to be saying that when a person constitutes a danger — real or potential — that person must be excluded and some form of control must be imposed on him or her. Society must be protected, and the institution serves this purpose by making sure that no one will threaten public tranquillity, the established order and the principles of social organization in a serious and sustained way. Thus, it is acknowledged that social equilibrium is delicate, fragile and vulnerable to dangers of this sort

— to unpredictable threats from people in certain categories. For a person who does not conform to society's basic rules, a variety of sanctions are possible, going as far as exclusion from the social environment through placement in a totalitarian institution. In sum, all three groups accept the psychiatric institution as one of a number of ways of controlling a person categorized as dangerous. While each group has a different threshold of tolerance, the principle persists across group lines and could be observed in the analysis. In the range of possibilities for excluding a person, the psychiatric institution constitutes an acceptable solution for all three groups.

7.1.2 The Concept of Work

People gain social value, a reason for being, and a justification of their existence within their environment through working, through being useful and productive. In sum, work lends harmony to social relations. People who manage to remain in the labour market even while deviating from social norms will gain recognition and acceptance more easily than those who, perhaps not by their own choice, boycott this principle or do not adhere to this rule.

The three groups of participants upheld the intrinsic value of work. For them, the question of excluding or not excluding an individual or a category of individuals was an important one. Leaders in society are often judged by their actions; thus, when it comes to judging another category of people, the same principle can be used to justify exclusion if these people do not contribute to building the social order through their work. Individual contribution through work is a major element in establishing personal worth, so that working constitutes a significant form of social integration. Even for those who end up being institutionalized, recognition and acceptance, both inside and outside the institution, will vary according to their integration into the productive world and their attitude to work. In sum, the evidence about participants' views of work lends credence to John Kenneth Galbraith's thesis that we have reached the point of identification with the technological and industrial era and that "normal" people want to adapt to the system. Exclusion awaits those who do not adhere to this rule.[1]

7.1.3 The Lack of Participation by "Deviants" in Responsibility for Their Care

None of the participants mentioned the possibility of excluded individuals playing an active role. What is their opinion? What is their version of events? Why did they commit such acts? Are they in favour of the idea of being sent to a psychiatric institution or not? In the interviews, no mention can be found of the principle of participation by the actors directly concerned during the process of exclusion.

This observation corroborates statistics on the rate of involuntary confinement in psychiatric institutions in New Brunswick; if that is the public attitude, it is hardly surprising that about 60 per cent of admissions are involuntary. The individual who is "at fault" commits acts; the group assesses their seriousness and decides on an appropriate penalty. This judgement — social and not personal — is the process that sets in motion the machinery of involuntary hospitalization (community, doctors, specialists, and so forth). Individuals "entrust" their actions to the arbitrary standard of the norm; the group judges and penalizes some individual actions.

When the group rejects an action or even an attitude, the next step is to take the individual in hand at public expense but at the price of individual freedom. Someone who doesn't internalize social norms has to suffer the consequences. As Robert and Françoise Castel and Anne Lovell have written:

Admirers of this sort of "democracy" generally neglect to point out that the aim is usually to achieve consensus, peacefully if possible, by force if necessary. The ideal would be a self-regulated system based on internalized controls, with each individual assuming responsibility for his own behaviour and for reproving deviant behaviour in his fellows.[2]

7.1.4 The Institution and "Treatment"

The idea of institutional therapy rarely arose in the interviews. There was no mention in the analysed discourse of the help that the institution could provide or its positive contribution to reestablishing the individual. What people say about the psychiatric institution leads to the conclusion that it is regarded more as an instrument of control than as a form of aid, assistance or care that can be provided to those who are committed there. Neither the institution nor psychiatric personnel are part of the *help-care* network as observed by the three groups. When people cannot be helped or cared for, they are treated. Thus, *treatment* becomes a synonym for confinement and control, for the benefit of the collectivity, while *help* is considered beneficial to the individual.

In all three ethnic groups, the fact that the terms *institution* and *mental* were closely associated could be observed. This observation is worth emphasizing and could be a subject for further research. Does this juxtaposition recur in the interviews simply by contagion, or is there an unconscious significance to the association of these two words by the participants? In the light of this question, how should the following statement by an inmate be interpreted: "If they keep me here [in the psychiatric hospital] much longer, I'll go crazy"? Can we carry the reasoning to the point of saying that the totalitarian institution is "mental" and, by contagion, draws people who stay there into the same category?

Our analysis showed that in the interviews, the institution is still regarded as playing the role that initially justified its existence in the sixteenth century: maintaining the social order, segregating madness and putting away certain categories of people. Dismissed by society, these people are taken in hand by a palliative institution that is medical in approach and totalitarian in character. It is in this sense that Christian Delacampagne has called the institution a "chance occurrence in the whole process by which psychiatry has taken society in hand."

A threefold role for the psychiatric institution emerges from this discussion. First of all, participants presented it as an instrument for protecting and rehabilitating the individual. According to the interviews, however, this role is a kind of façade, a pretense whose contradictions are revealed by the analysis. Participants also saw the institution as a means of protecting society against these same individuals. And finally, it is a form of medical-social "treatment" that takes different directions depending on the beliefs of the era (steam, electricity, drugs, and so forth).

Today, even if psychiatric institutions are closing their doors, their influence on society remains as great as ever. The practice of psychiatry and the "treatment" of people no longer take place within four walls; instead, on the pretext of prevention, they run through the entire organization of society, which threatens to become totalitarian as a result. In this sense, the walls of the asylum are becoming normative rather than physical.

7.1.5 Conformity: Individual and Social Responsibility

A conception of the internalization of norms by the individual also emerges from the interviews. It is implied that individuals are capable of integrating and conforming to social norms. Under certain circumstances, they deserve to be helped or cared for. If these palliatives and community remedies do not work, or if the individual does not deserve them, then the methods become more drastic and control becomes stricter: the institution and treatment.

Of course, nonconformity is accepted in some cases; examples are the mentally retarded and the rich. For the first group, however, special schools—places of apprenticeship and control— are built. For the second, it seems that their social status helps them escape the sanctions that apply to ordinary mortals. This could explain the fact that there are so few representatives of the liberal professions and the wealthy classes in psychiatric institutions.

7.1.6 The Forms of Madness

Three forms of madness emerge from the interviews:
• Social madness: here the mad person plays a role that is accepted or even valued within society. This form is most evident in the Acadian group, and is illustrated by the example of "Joe Fou", "Henri Fou" and the like. Mad people of this sort have a certain social usefulness.
• Tolerated deviance: some mentally ill people, although categorized as abnormal, continue to live in society in a more or less marginal fashion. The mentally retarded are a good illustration of this phenomenon. People who are "depressed" or "disturbed" or "have a case of nerves" also fit in this category.
• Dangerous madness: this category comprises people who are considered incapable of controlling their actions and are accepted by society only if they are institutionalized, primarily because of the danger they represent. There is a certain code of moral judgement that applies to the acts of these deviants so that there are some who are tolerated and others who are locked up. Most of the time, it is people in this category who are hospitalized involuntarily.

Although the Irish, Acadians and Loyalists all maintain the same categories, the three groups do not necessarily place the same people in each category. We will see further on that norms vary and each group has its own perception of social, tolerated and dangerous madness. Nevertheless, the categories appear to be universal for the population under study.

7.2 POINTS OF DIVERGENCE AMONG THE THREE GROUPS UNDER STUDY

In comparing the three sets of interviews, we also find some differences that are worth pointing out.

7.2.1 How the Groups Relate to Deviants

While the concepts of *help*, *care* and *treatment* are common to the three groups, the idea of *help* and *care* through traditional networks of assistance assumed major significance in the interviews with the Acadians while the other two groups gave it relatively less weight.

Among the Loyalists in particular, there appears to be a more categorical rejection of deviants. Loyalists entrust them to experts and the institution more systematically and arbitrarily, and are more inclined to associate deviance with danger and with the forms of control needed to prevent such danger or keep it in check. In sum, the question for them is not curing individuals but preserving the social order that these individuals threaten, and they place more emphasis on the social order than on individual well-being. There is little concern with the needs of mad people or the reasons behind their condition. The relationship with deviants becomes more impersonal, distant, through third parties. The Irish maintain that the family must have a role in treating the mentally ill person; it is the family, with the help of experts, that should decide whether the person should be committed. This idea of family involvement is not found among the Loyalists.

The Acadians mentioned the priest, the family and friends as forming part of the basic process of therapy and assigned each of them a share of the responsibility when the time comes to decide whether or not to commit the individual to a psychiatric institution. In sketching the history of psychiatry in Quebec, Robert Mayer and Henri Dorvil expressed an opinion that tallied with these observations: "In French Canada, mad people have a certain place in traditional society, while in English Canada, no one shows much interest in them."[3]

Thus, the place of the mad person differs from group to group. Among the Acadians, mad people can still have a certain traditional role; the Irish have a greater tendency to isolate them in the family or the institution; while for the Loyalists, the institution is clearly the solution of choice.

7.2.2 Dangerous Madness

When there is danger, all three groups choose the institutional solution, but the concept of danger does not have the same significance for the different groups. Thus, analysis of the interviews with the Loyalists revealed that most of the categories of deviants were considered dangerous. Both the Irish and the Acadians appear to have a higher threshold of tolerance, and in both these groups people are referred to the traditional network of care and help before being sent to the institution.

Thus, each group has its own scale of tolerance for deviance. Among the Acadians, danger centres on the concept of *trouble*. A dangerous person is one who disturbs or threatens the peace by causing trouble, and it is hard for Acadians to accept such a "troubled" person. For the Irish, the medical approach plays a more central role, and they use the term *mental* to designate sick people, who are committed if they cannot be kept in the community. The Loyalists use the same term, but they use it twice as often in an equivalent amount of text and they constantly associate it with the institution. Thus, the Irish are different from the Loyalists in their family and social concern for deviants. These relationships can be summarized as follows:

• The Acadians interpret deviance on the basis of events in daily life, try to discover its causes, and reject dangerous people who are "troubled" or cause "trouble."

• The Irish are ashamed of the mentally ill and hide them. This may be a reflection of a degree of social guilt or else a solution to the dilemma of rejection or responsibility.

• The Loyalists openly entrust dangerous deviants to professional and institutional services. This rejection applies both to people who are actually dangerous and to those who are potentially so. Loyalists resort to the institutional solution more quickly than the other two groups.

7.2.3 How the Groups Relate to the Institution and Experts

A variety of relationships to the institution emerge from these observations and comparisons. For all three groups, the psychiatric institution appears to be a solution that is necessary for the functioning of society and the social, political and economic order. In the interviews, none of the three groups completely rejected the institution.

Dr. Alex Richman has tried to establish a relationship between physical distance from the institution and rate of involuntary hospitalization. However, another form of distance between each of the three groups and the institution can be posited:

• The Acadians see the institution as coming after the traditional network of help (represented by neighbours and friends) and care (represented by the priest, the doctor and finally the institution).

• The Irish express their concern for mad people by hiding them, then by entrusting them to a community care network (home, doctor, family), and finally by committing them.

• The Loyalists demonstrate a much closer equivalence in the interviews between confinement in a psychiatric institution and deviance; this solution is nearer and more immediate.

It was also in the city with the greatest concentration of Loyalists that the first psychiatric institution was built. This institution appears to play a larger role in the "treatment" of deviants for the Loyalists than for the other two groups. It should also be noted that the rate of involuntary hospitalization is greatest in Saint John. At the same time, it is worth mentioning that Acadian society established other mechanisms to exclude its deviants, such as sale of the poor at auction and use of the Tracadie leper-hospital.[4] Little study of these mechanisms has been done.

These observations, based on content analysis of the interviews, indicate that the second hypothesis partly stands up to analysis, in the sense that each of the groups demonstrates a different perception of the network of services offered and the use of the institution. We saw in chapter 5 that the reasons mentioned for admission were very different from group to group (see especially table 14, p. 91). These observations about proximity

Figure 15
Systems of Expertise by Ethnic Group

Ethnic Group	Primary System	Secondary System	Tertiary System
Acadians	Family and friends (help)	Clergy and doctors (care)	Institution (treatment)
Irish	Family and friends (help, hiding)	Community care system (hiding)	Institution (treatment)
Loyalists	Institution (treatment)	Institution (treatment)	Institution (treatment)

are a kind of complement to the statistical analysis, especially in this regard.

7.3 PROFILE OF THE THREE GROUPS UNDER STUDY

It emerges from studying the interviews that the three groups' conceptions of deviance come together under certain headings and diverge significantly under others. The points of convergence centre on the themes of danger to society and the need for the institution as an instrument of repression and control. Among the points of divergence are the interpretation of the term *dangerous* and, as a result, the degree of use of the institution for people categorized in that way (see figure 15).

NOTES

1. See John Kenneth Galbraith, *The New Industrial State* (London: Andre Deutsch, 1972), chapter 12.
2. Robert Castel, Françoise Castel, and Anne Lovell, *The Psychiatric Society* (New York: Columbia University Press, 1982), p. 312.
3. Robert Mayer and Henri Dorvil, "La Psychiatrie au Québec: réalité d'hier, pratique d'aujourd'hui," in Association Canadienne de Sociologie et d'Anthropologie de Langue Française, *Rapport du Colloque* (Montreal: Editions Saint-Martin, 1982), p. 116.
4. See Mary Jane Losier and Céline Pinet, *Les enfants de Lazare* (Moncton: Editions d'Acadie, 1987).

Conclusion

*I have found that in
psychiatric hospitals madness
is actually quite rare.*

—David Cooper

In this study, an attempt has been made to present a profile of national oppression in psychiatric treatment in New Brunswick, concentrating especially on the situation of one minority, the Acadians, in comparison with two other ethnic groups, the Irish and the Loyalists. As the analysis took shape, a number of working hypotheses were proposed. The three approaches that were used and the results obtained are summed up and brought together in the following pages.

Who is mad?

Legislative terminology, specialists and the people who were interviewed for this study all seem unable to define madness and describe and pinpoint those who should be covered by mental health legislation or hospitalized in psychiatric institutions. A "danger to oneself or others" is a constantly recurring theme, but while it is conceivable that a "mad" person could be dangerous, no systematic one-to-one correspondence can be established between the two concepts.

In short, the definition of madness would appear to be arbitrary, relative and dependent on the interests of particular groups in society. It is obvious that normality and the acceptable limits of deviance are defined by certain kinds of specialists and interested parties. Thus, it can be asked whether the authorities in charge of the process of involuntary hospitalization are impartial and what kind of power is wielded by the institutions involved in this process. The well-being and safety of the individual or the community are always cited as central concerns, but it is not always easy to verify that this is so.

Whose interests does psychiatry serve?

Following on the questions raised about madness, it may be noted that psychiatry as a science is only vaguely defined, and the impasse it is facing at present is at least in part the result of that vagueness. The direction psychiatry and the system that supports it (which includes doctors, the police, social workers and others) are taking needs to be reassessed. Involuntary admission is but a sign, a symptom, rather than the problem itself. Understanding this, it has been possible to go back to the origins of asylums, to reflect on their ideological as well as their psychiatric function, and to raise the question of political and cultural influences on psychiatry in particular historical contexts. As David Cooper has noted, "politics borrows the mask of psychiatry to do violence to people."[1] In short, what distinguishes mad people is not that they are mad but that they are held in restraint; people are shut away in psychiatric institutions — with supporting diagnoses — and thus become members of that group of deviants which is considered mad.

This study has revealed a number of disturbing facts about New Brunswick psychiatric institutions and the people who make them work, in the areas of reasons for admission, length of stay, and the medical and psychiatric treatment of deviants. We have looked at confinement in psychiatric institutions as a response in western societies over the past three centuries to illnesses suffered by individuals and manifested in an individual way. Writing about the nineteenth century, Michel Foucault has said that this method of treatment "became ever more urgent but increasingly difficult, increasingly ineffective."[2] On the whole, the method of treatment has changed little. It still involves institutionalization, with reliance on specialists and legal support, as the solution for cases of deviance. It has been applied in New Brunswick to the detriment of social groups of all kinds that refuse to conform to the prevailing social order. Since minorities are by definition nonconformist, the Acadians, as we have demonstrated, have suffered the most from the way psychiatry functions.

Psychiatry in English

In New Brunswick, psychiatry is practised primarily in English, which means that many psychiatrists who are English in language and outlook have been entrusted with therapeutic reponsibilities that take them beyond their own cultural experience. An individual's mother tongue is an essential medium for the expression of her or his feelings; non-English speakers who are obliged to speak English are already a step removed from those feelings and perhaps cut off from the essence of their being — the source of authenticity and therefore of individual and collective health. The psychiatric treatment to which Acadians are subjected, in a context where they are made to suffer for their minority status, amounts to the virtual dissolution of their collective identity.

Thus, in the area of mental health, national oppression is perpetuated and reproduced through what Jean-Paul Sartre has called "seriality." Seriality is but one facet of the disintegration characteristic of our age. It is the opposite of a fused group, the only basis on which collective goals can be reached and effective responsibility for institutions that provide the framework of everyday life can be taken.

Normalization through treatment

Normalization is the process through which psychiatrists become agents of the prevailing social order, a kind of cultural police force whose task is to ensure that the norms of the majority are respected. We have seen, for example, that, proportionally speaking, Acadians are subjected to psychiatric treatment in significantly greater numbers than the English.

The enforcement of majority norms cannot be carried out in the same way for the Acadians as for nonconformist English groups. For English speakers, even deviant social behaviour and activities are part of the same cultural universe as the norm. To be sure, this does not mean that the transition between one form of behaviour and another is not painful or that it does not cause a real disturbance in mental structures. In the case of Acadians, however, we are dealing with a transition from one cultural universe to another. Such a process carries a risk of denaturing those involved, and this is usually what occurs. Psychiatric treatment can only hasten this process and carry it to its logical conclusion.

Just as dreams are a distillation of expectations and desires that are unfulfilled in our waking hours, so illness is a distillation of an overall imbalance in the individual. The focus shifts continually back and forth between the collective and individual planes. The collective experience of national oppression affects the individual consciousness. Illness is merely an echo, calling out like a cry of despair and pointing to the social and political causes of the problem. It urges us to look to these unseen causes that produce diseases in ways that the power games of the elite never allow us to see.

Forms of intolerance and types of societies

Minorities are by definition groups that the majority merely tolerates. In times of crisis, minorities experience the contradictions of society as a whole with added intensity, while in calm periods, their behaviour is subject to social controls that leave them little room to manoeuvre. Excluded from the political and economic spheres, they have very few opportunities to give their energies a social direction and develop their own world view.

The Irish keep certain kinds of rejection hidden at home. Rejecting, watching over and hiding, all at the same time — this appears to be a way in which they are able to come to terms with misfortunes of this sort.

The Acadians seem to be afraid of trouble and want to avoid situations of conflict. The social consensus is maintained by getting rid of and silencing people whose behaviour betrays the existence of social disorders. This strategy has negative implications for the Acadians' political prospects. Agitators are rejected because they are "troubled," and troubled people are sent to psychiatrists. It is a paradoxical situation. There is a need for leaders who know and understand Acadian society. However, when such people become socially and politically aware and bring certain issues to a head, they are taken care of by the psychiatric system and Acadian self-censorship.

Very early on, religious morality and a sense of civic duty forced the Acadians into submissive behaviour that does not allow for conflict. It is as if to engage in conflict were un-Acadian. Avoiding situations of conflict requires a great deal of agility. In this context, anyone who makes a commitment and polarizes contradictions is seen as an unreasonable person, as someone talking nonsense. Neutrality, rooted in the Acadians' collective stance, comes across as a constant in Acadian culture that would be almost impossible to eliminate. The other extreme, social and political involvement, is virtually equated with madness. "Woe betide the man through whom scandal comes": nowhere has the truth of this saying been as fully borne out as in Acadia. Whoever dares to provoke the prevailing social order runs the risk of expulsion, either into physical exile or into madness.

With very few exceptions, the Acadian way of thinking does not allow anyone to express major differences. Any attempt to do so is quickly labelled, disposed of as deviant and excluded. We can see this as a case of double repression — internal self-repression, similar to what Roy Preiswerk has described as self-colonization, and the sociopolitical repression spoken of earlier.

The Loyalists are categorical and firm when it comes to deviants, entrusting them without hesitation to institutions and specialists. However, according to our analysis of the interviews, this is not because the Loyalists have confidence in the treatment provided. Rather, it is an attempt to suppress social contradictions. Madness can have its own territory, its own government: what counts is public safety, public order and ideological conformity.

The outlook for Acadia

Acadians are responding to the process of alienation outlined in this study in a number of ways. One such response is a movement for autonomy that represents a real break with the *bon-ententiste* approach of the old elites, whose purely reformist goals never touched the institutions that guaranteed the reproduction of the social foundations of majority power.

Only this movement for autonomy can change the health situation without intensifying the oppression of the Acadian community. The main purpose of autonomy is to recreate a truly Acadian social fabric with political, economic and ideological manifestations. The health situation will inevitably be affected by this process. Achieving autonomy means becoming a healthy people that has broken the chains of dependence and is moving towards a future based on a collective vision developed by and for Acadians.

NOTES

1. "Qui sont les fous?", interview with David Cooper, *L'Education* no. 332 (November 10, 1977), p. 34.
2. Michel Foucault, *Histoire de la folie à l'âge classique* (Paris: Gallimard, 1972), p. 424.

Bibliography

Bardin, Laurence. *L'Analyse de contenu*. Paris: Presses Universitaires de France, 1977.

Barel, Yves. *La Marginalité sociale*. Paris: Presses Universitaires de France, 1982.

Bastide, Roger. The *Sociology of Mental Disorder*. London: Routledge and Kegan Paul, 1972.

Basaglia, Franco. *La Majorité déviante*. Paris: Union Générale d'Editions, 1976.

Bélanger, Paul R., and Saint-Pierre, Céline. "Dépendance économique, subordination politique et oppression nationale." *Sociologie et sociétés* no. 10 (October 1978), pp. 123-47.

Bettelheim, Bruno, and Karlin, Daniel. Un *autre regard sur la folie*. Paris: Stock & Plus, 1979.

Boudreau, Francoise. *De l'asile à la santé mentale*. Montreal: Editions Saint-Martin, 1984.

Bozzini, L., et al., eds. *Médecine et société, les années 1980*. Montreal: Editions Saint-Martin, 1984.

Braen, André. *La Santé au Nouveau-Brunswick*. Moncton: Société des Acadiens du Nouveau-Brunswick, 1981.

Canada. Statistics Canada. *One of Eight: Mental Illness in Canada* . Ottawa: Supply and Services, 1981.

Cassen, Bernard. "La langue anglaise comme véhicule de l'impérialisme culturel." *L'homme et la société*, nos. 47-50 (Jan.-Dec. 1978), pp. 95-104.

Castel, Robert. La *gestion des risques*. Paris: Minuit, 1981.

Castel, Robert; Castel, Françoise; and Lovell, Anne. *The Psychiatric Society*. New York: Columbia University Press, 1982.

Chen, Dorothy. *Historical Facts on the Provincial Hospital.*. Mimeo. June 1967.

Chesler, Phyllis. *Women and Madness*. New York: Avon Books, 1973.

Cooper, David. *Psychiatry and Anti-Psychiatry*. London: Tavistock Publications Ltd., 1967.

Cushing, Travis. "Some History of Mental Health in New Brunswick." In *Report on the Provincial Conference on Mental Health Held by the New Brunswick Division of the Canadian Mental Health Association, Memramcook Institute, November 12 - 14, 1976*. Mental Health/New Brunswick and Canadian Mental Health Association, n.d.

Delacampagne, Christian. *Antipsychiatrie, les voies du sacré*. Paris: Grasset, 1974.

Delacampagne, Christian. *Figures de l'oppression*. Paris: Presses Universitaires de France, 1977.

Devereux, Georges. *Essais d'ethnopsychiatrie générale*. Paris: Gallimard, 1970.

Donzelot, Jacques. *The Policing of Families*. New York: Pantheon Books, 1979.

Dumond, G.J. "French Canadian Descendance and Mental Health: An Exploratory Study." Master's thesis, School of Social Work, Smith College, Northampton, Mass., 1980.

Durkheim, Emile. *The Division of Labour in Society*. New York: Free Press of Glencoe, 1964.

Duvignaud, Jean. *L'anomie: hérésie et subversion*. Paris: Anthropos, 1973.

Even, Alain. "Le Territoire pilote du Nouveau-Brunswick ou les blocages culturels au développement économique." Doctoral thesis, Faculté de droit et de Sciences économiques, Université de Rennes, 1970.

Fanon, Frantz. *The Wretched of the Earth*. New York: Grove Press, 1966.

Fellow, Robert. *Researching Your Ancestors in New Brunswick*. Fredericton, n.d..

Foucault, Michel. *The Birth of the Clinic: An Archaeology of Medical Perception*. London: Tavistock Press, Ltd., 1973.

Foucault, Michel. *Histoire de la folie à l'âge classique*. Paris: Gallimard, 1972.

Foucault, Michel., *Madness and Civilization: A History of Insanity in the Age of Reason*. London: Tavistock Publications Ltd., 1965.

Galbraith, John Kenneth. *The New Industrial State*. London: Andre Deutsch, 1972.

Gentis, Roger. *Les murs de l'asile*. Paris: Maspero, 1970.

Godin, Pierre. *Cinq ans de trop*. Petit-Rocher, N.B., 1971.

Goffman, Erving. *Asylums*. Garden City, N.Y.: Anchor Books, 1961.

Gove, Walter R., and Tudor, Jeannette F. "Adult Sex Role and Mental Illness." *American Journal of Sociology* 78:812-35.

Hughes, Charles, et al. *People of Cove and Woodlot*. New York: Basic Books, 1960.

Illich, Ivan. *Medical Nemesis*. Toronto: McClelland and Stewart, 1975.

Kirsh, Sharon. *Unemployment, Its Impact on Body and Soul.*. Toronto: Canadian Mental Health Association, 1983.

Laing, R.D. *The Politics of Experience*. New York: Pantheon Books, 1967.

Laing, R.D., and Cooper, David. *Reason and Violence: A Decade of Sartre's Philosophy*. London: Tavistock Publications, 1964.

Laing, R.D, and Esterton, A. *Sanity, Madness and the Family: Families of Schizophrenics*. New York: Basic Books, 1971.

LeBlanc, Raymond. *Cri de terre*. Moncton: Editions d'Acadie, 1972.

Leighton, A.H. *Caring for Mentally Ill People: Psychological and Social Barriers in Historical Context*. Cambridge: At the University Press, 1982.

Lenoir, René. *Les exclus*. Paris: Seuil, 1974.

Liégeois, J. P. "Le Discours de l'ordre; pouvoir public et minorité culturelle." *Esprit* no. 5 (May 1980), pp. 17-43.

Losier, Mary Jane and Pinet, Céline. Les enfants de Lazare. Editions d'Acadie, 1987.

Maillet, Antonine. *Pélagie* . Garden City, N.Y.: Doubleday, 1982.

Mannoni, Maud. *Le psychiatre, son "fou" et la psychanalyse.* Paris: Seuil, 1970.

Martin, Chester. "The Loyalists in New Brunswick." *Ontario Historical Society* 30 (1934): 165-66.

Mayer, Robert, and Dorvil, Henri. "La Psychiatrie au Québec: réalité d'hier, pratique d'aujourd'hui." In Association Canadienne de Sociologie et d'Anthropologie de Langue Française, *Rapport du Colloque* (Montreal: Editions Saint-Martin, 1982).

Nadeau, Robert. "Michel Foucault ou le développement impitoyable." *Critère* no. 13 (March 1976).

New Brunswick. Department of Health. *Annual Reports,* 1956-1981.

New Brunswick. Legislative Assembly. *Report of the Medical Superintendent for 1851.*

O'Neill, John. "Decolonization and the Ideal Speech Community: Some Issues in the Theory and Practice of Communicative Competence." In *Critical Theory and Public Life,* edited by John Forester. Cambridge, Mass.: MIT Press, 1985.

O'Neill, John, "Le Langage et la décolonisation." *Sociologies et Sociétés* 6, no. 2: 54.

Pagé, J. C. *Les fous crient au secours.* Témoignage d'un ex-patient de St-Jean-de-Dieu. Montreal: Editions du Jour, 1961.

Paquet-Deehy, Anne, et al. "Les femmes sont-elles plus malades que les hommes?" Unpublished paper delivered in Halifax, June 1981.

Paradis, A., et al. *Essais pour une préhistoire de la psychiatrie au Canada (1800-885).* Recherches et théories no. 15. Montreal and Trois-Rivières: Université du Quebec, 1977.

Preiswerk, Roy. *Le savoir et le faire.* Paris: Presses Universitaires de France, 1975.

"Qui sont les fous?" Interview with David Cooper. *L'Education* no. 332 (November 10, 1977), p. 34.

Reversy, J.F. *La Folie dans la rue.* Toulouse: Privat, 1978.

Riesman, David. *The Lonely Crowd.* New Haven: Yale University Press, 1961.

Riley, Rodney, and Richman, Alex. "Involuntary Hospitalization to Mental and Psychiatric Hospitals in Canada." Unpublished paper delivered in Winnipeg, September 1981.

Robichaud, Jean-Bernard. *La santé des francophones.* 3 vols. Moncton: Editions d'Acadie, 1985.

Robichaud, Louis. "The Acadian Outlook (1)." In *French Canada Today,* edited by C.F. MacRae. Sackville, N.B.: Mount Allison University, 1961.

Rothman, David. *The Discovery of the Asylum.* Boston: Little, Brown and Co., 1971.

Roy, Michel. *L'Acadie perdue.* Montreal: Québec/Amérique, 1978.

St-Amand, Néré. "L'Internement en institution psychiatrique: ses rapports avec l'origine ethnique et le processus d'industrialisation." Doctoral thesis, Université de Nice, 1983.

St-Amand, Néré. "La Santé mentale au Nouveau-Brunswick: bref historique et observations." *Revue de l'Université de Moncton* 13, no. 3 (1980): 167-85.

Satir, Virginia. *Conjoint Family Therapy: A Guide to Theory and Technique.* Palo Alto, Calif.: Science and Behavior Books, 1964.

Sirois, R., and Fortier, S. *Problèmes linguistiques de l'hôpital psychiatrique de Campbellton.* Unpublished study presented to the New Brunswick Department of Health, December 1981.

Stanley, Della Margaret Maude. *Au service de deux peuples.* Moncton: Editions d'Acadie, 1977.

Sow, Alfa Ibrahim. *Anthropological Structures of Madness in Black Africa.* New York: International Universities Press, 1980.

Stiker, Henri-Jacques. *Corps infirmes et societes.* Paris: Aubier, 1982.

Szasz, Thomas. *Ideology and Insanity: Essays on the Psychiatric Dehumanization of Man.* Garden City, N.Y.: Anchor Books, 1970.

Szasz, Thomas. *Law, Liberty and Psychiatry: An Enquiry into the Social Uses of Mental Health Practices.* New York: Macmillan, 1963.

Szasz, Thomas. *The Theology of Medicine.* Baton Rouge: Louisiana State University Press, 1977.

Tremblay, Marc-Adélard, and Gold, Gérald Louis. *Communautés et culture: éléments pour une ethnologie du Canada français.* Montreal: HRW, 1973.